P9-DFJ-219

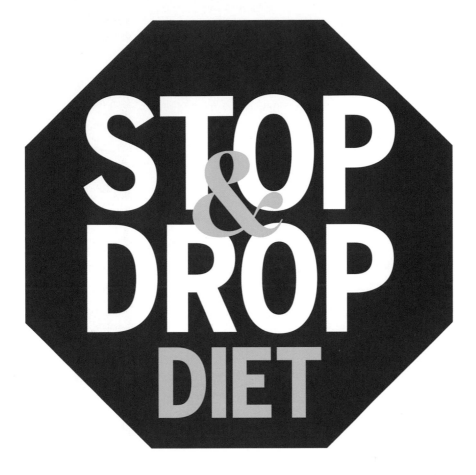

STOP & DROP DIET

Lose up to 5 Pounds in 5 Days

LIZ VACCARIELLO

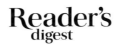

The Reader's Digest Association, Inc.
New York NY/Montreal

A READER'S DIGEST BOOK

Copyright © 2015 The Reader's Digest Association, Inc.

Food photographs by Ali Blumenthal, Dan Roberts, Jim Wieland, Grace Natoli Sheldon, and Mark Derse

Tester photographs by Steve Vaccariello

Library of Congress Cataloging-in-Publication Data
Vaccariello, Liz.
  Stop & drop diet / Liz Vaccariello
      pages cm
  Includes index.
    Summary: "*New York Times* bestselling author and *Reader's Digest*
editor-in-chief Liz Vaccariello presents the easiest diet ever, teaching you
how to stop eating unhealty versions of the foods you love and offering quick
and easy meals you can find or make anywhere you go using your favorite
everyday brand-name foods—so you can drop up to 5 pounds in 5 days!"
—Provided by publisher.
  ISBN 978-1-62145-260-7 (hardback) -- ISBN 978-1-62145-261-4 (epub)
1. Weight loss--Popular works. 2. Reducing diets--Popular works. 3.
Health--Popular works. 4. Nutrition--Popular works. I. Hermann, Mindy
G. II. Title. III. Title: Stop and drop diet.
  RM222.2.V257 2015
  613.2'5--dc23
                              2015026670

We are committed to both the quality of our products and the service we provide
to our customers. We value your comments, so please feel free to contact us.
        The Reader's Digest Association, Inc.
        Adult Trade Publishing
        44 South Broadway
        White Plains, NY 10601

For more Reader's Digest products and information, visit our website:
        www.rd.com

Printed in China

10 9 8 7 6 5 4 3 2 1

NOTE TO OUR READERS
The information in this book should not be substituted for, or used to alter, medical
therapy without your doctor's advice. For a specific health problem, consult your
physician for guidance.

Mention of specific companies, organizations, or authorities in this book does
not imply endorsement by the author or publisher, nor does mention of specific
companies, organizations, or authorities imply that they endorse this book, its
author, or the publisher. The brand-name products mentioned in this book are
trademarks or registered trademarks of their respective companies. Internet
addresses, telephone numbers, and product information given in this book were
accurate at the time it went to press.

Reader's Digest tested the diet with 10 readers and employees. Testers were not paid
to participate. How much weight you lose will vary depending on your gender, age,
and starting weight, plus what you typically eat and how much you exercise, among
many other factors. Even using the same program of diet and exercise, individual
results will vary. Losing 1 pound a day is not a typical result.

CONTENTS

Acknowledgments
THANK YOU

So many people made the *Stop & Drop Diet* possible that I hardly know where to begin.

Mindy Hermann scoured and searched, analyzed and organized the more than 700 foods in this book. Her deep knowledge and experience—not to mention patience and professionalism—are the heart of this book.

Likewise, Andrea Au Levitt shepherded the *Stop & Drop Diet* from budget to bookstore. She is an editor of many talents (extraordinary attention to detail among them), and I don't know how I'd produce a book without her.

Rebecca Simpson Steele is *Reader's Digest*'s photo director. She devoted hundreds of hours to planning and executing multiple food and product shoots—and produced the almost two dozen video shoots for our incredible online course. Her keen eye, her commitment to excellence, and her ability to "handle the talent" are all gifts I am thankful for every day.

Ali Blumenthal is *Reader Digest*'s photo assistant and helped with many aspects of the project. As an accomplished photographer in her own right, we counted on her to photograph the hundreds of packaged foods in the book. I am grateful for the endless hours Ali spent both in the studio and at her desk!

Many thanks also to the team at the *Taste of Home* photo studio, who helped us capture all the meal, restaurant, and recipe photos, especially Kerri Balliet, Sarah Thompson, Stephanie Marchese, and Ester Robards. And thanks to Catherine Cassidy for supporting this project in so many ways!

Lauren Gelman and Kelsey Kloss are the heart of *Reader's Digest*'s health team. As director, Lauren was instrumental in pulling together lessons and scripts for the *Stop & Drop Online Course*. Kelsey worked on almost every aspect of the product suite, writing, researching, organizing, checking, and rechecking.

It was with breathtaking grace and admirable fearlessness that Courtenay Smith jumped into her role masterminding the *Stop & Drop Online Course*. She is executive editor of *Reader's Digest* by day, but eye of the

Stop & Drop hurricane by night. I am abundantly grateful for all she does for our magazine, this product, and my spirit. Thank you for your candor, your wisdom, your tenacity, and your many many skills. I wouldn't dare do a book or tape a segment without you!

Of course, Courtenay's laser focus and commitment were possible because of the multitalented team on *Reader's Digest* that picked up the slack: Managing director of content operations and all around editorial wunderkind Kerrie Keegan; executive editor and the heart of so much of *Reader's Digest*, Barbara O'Dair; and creative director Dean Abatemarco, who never met a design he couldn't fix, a cover he couldn't improve.

Senior designer Gloria Tebelman saved the day in more ways than I can count. Her vision for the *Stop & Drop Diet* book cover, her design of Part Three, her production of the online course graphics . . . everything is just better thanks to Gloria.

Reader's Digest's book department has a deep well of talent. Fearless leader Debra Polansky, editorial director Jim Menick, art director George McKeon, managing editor Lorraine Burton, master marketers and salespeople Kim Gray, Veronica Gonzalez, and Nancy Taylor. Harold Clarke, you believed from the very beginning. I thank you and miss you.

In consumer marketing, I thank Leslie Doty, Valerie Federice, Karen Berner, Jamele Polk, Jess Wesley, Mary Melian, and the rest of their talented teams.

Special thanks also to the small army of copyeditors, proofreaders, fact-checkers, food shoppers, designers, and other helpers without which this book could not have happened: Susan Hindman, Mary Jane DeFroscia, Nancee Adams-Taylor, Shara Beitch, Alyssa Jung, Brooke Wanser, Will Sabbagh, Drew Salvatore, Sierra Rinaldi, Claire Nowak, Elizabeth Tunnicliffe, Wayne Morrison, and John Cassidy.

Pauli Cohen, Sabrina Strauss, and the Goodman PR team, you're an author's best friend.

Hugs to my dear friends at *The Doctors*: Jay McGraw, Travis Stork, Shannon Hunt, Andrea McKinnon, Patricia Ciano, Jeff Hudson, Keegan Heise, and team.

And a huge shout-out to my fellow Stop & Drop testers: Nora Healy, Donna Lindskog, Angela Mastrantuono, Carol Maymudes, Diane Rohan, Eileen Supran, Karen Woytach, Joe and Kim Gray, and Randi Zelkin.

Adrienne Farr, where would I be without you?

Steve, Olivia, and Sophia, what would I do?

And of course none of this is possible without the woman with the plan, Bonnie Kintzer. Thank you for being a leader, mentor, and all-around inspiration.

Introduction
HOW TO USE THIS BOOK

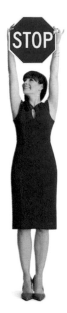

I've written several diet books over the past few years, each attempting to help readers solve the seemingly intractable problem of weight loss. Each time, at least one person writes to me here at Reader's Digest or contacts me on social media to say something to the effect of, "If your last diet really worked, why do you need to write another one?"

My standard answer is this: While I always try to make my diets user-friendly and accessible, not every diet works for everyone. Some people want to be told exactly what to eat from day to day; others just want a few general principles to follow. Some people are happy to cook every meal; others find that impossibly daunting. Some people have 100 or more pounds to lose; others merely a few. Some people are ready to change their whole lifestyle; others are only willing to make a few small tweaks.

Personally, I've always taken a health-focused approach to weight loss, drilling down into the latest science to attack specific physiological challenges that hurt health and lead to weight gain. In my book *Flat Belly Diet!*, for instance, I focused on the amazing nutrient—monounsaturated fatty acids, or MUFAs—that can target deadly belly fat. Then, scientists uncovered a dozen other fat releasers, the basis for my book *The Digest Diet*. Most recently, I wrote the *21-Day Tummy Diet* to share the groundbreaking new research about foods that simultaneously shrink your belly and soothe common gastrointestinal issues. Thousands of readers have succeeded in losing weight and improving their overall health following these diets.

But if I'm honest, some of these diets required a good bit of work—shopping for specific foods and the occasional hard-to-find or expensive ingredient (I'm looking at you, flaxseed oil!). Many people just want to get the pounds off fast. And they want to learn easy strategies so they can make better decisions throughout their day, no matter where they are or what their goals. They don't want to count calories or fat grams. They don't want to cook one thing for themselves and something different for the rest of the family. And they don't want to give up their favorite foods. They want a diet, a way to eat, that fits seamlessly into their busy lifestyle. And they want the weight to drop off and stay off.

That's why I wrote this book. Is it possible to create a diet that works for each and every dieter? No. But I believe the Stop & Drop Diet comes pretty darn close. That's because it delivers the two things all dieters want: (1) fast results and (2) maximum flexibility. Plus, it shows you how to *stop* eating unhealthy versions of the foods you love so you can *drop* the weight fast.

How the Book Is Organized

The book is organized into three parts: Part One explains the basic principles of the diet. Part Two *is* the diet. Part Three presents the wide world of foods so you can make smart Stop & Drop choices forever, no matter where you go.

In Part One, I'll describe how we designed the Stop & Drop Diet with the twin goals of fast results and maximum flexibility in mind. First, you'll learn *why* you need to stop before you eat or buy foods, *what* you need to stop doing, and *how* stopping gives you time to check in with your body and make smart food choices. You'll learn how to spot hidden calories so you can stop eating unhealthy versions of your usual meals. Then you'll see how making smart food choices throughout the day can add up to big calorie savings—enough for you to drop a pound a day or even more. Finally, you'll discover just what makes the Stop & Drop Diet so easy to follow—the inclusion of everyday brand-name foods; the flexibility to eat out, grab and go, or make your own; the ability to mix and match meals from multiple calorie levels.

In Part Two, you'll find the Stop & Drop meals. This is the 3-week diet plan. This is what makes the Stop & Drop Diet different from other calorie-comparison guides. If you're eager to get started, you can jump right here to see the wide variety of foods you will choose from on the 3-week diet. The Stop & Drop Diet has three different calorie levels: Kickstart, which gives you 1200 calories per day; Steady Loss, 1600 calories per day; and Maintain, 2000 calories per day. As the name implies, Kickstart is designed to jump-start weight loss; we recommend that most people begin with this level for a week. Then, to avoid boredom, weight loss plateaus, and other common dieting challenges, we suggest switching to the Steady Loss plan until you reach your goal weight, after which you go on to the Maintain phase.

But you don't have to follow this exact timetable; you can easily customize the Stop & Drop Diet to fit your goals and lifestyle. If you want to lose weight for your reunion in a month, for instance, you may opt to stay on Kickstart for up to 3 weeks (though you'll see that we don't recommend staying on it indefinitely, for a number of reasons). On the other hand, if you are very active, 1200 calories may not be enough for you, in which case you can do Kickstart for just a few days, then move up to Steady Loss. You get the idea.

This is not a Day 1, Day 2, Day 3 eating plan. For each stage of the diet, we've laid out about 20 breakfasts, 20 lunches, and 20 dinners. You decide what to eat! And keep in mind that you can eat foods from earlier phases throughout the diet. If you really like Kickstart Breakfast #17 (Greek yogurt with berries and granola), for instance, you can keep having that for breakfast throughout your Steady Loss or even your Maintain phase. I did just that myself! You never have to force yourself to eat something you don't like; if there are meals on the list that don't appeal to you, simply skip them. No matter how you put the meals together, you'll be making smarter choices and you'll be losing weight.

All the meals in Part Two were created with foods featured in Part Three, often rounded out with fruits or vegetables and sometimes including a beverage or a dessert. Part Three is designed to help you make the smartest food choices wherever you are. For each type of food, we list the unhealthy versions you should *stop* eating—those that are highest in calories and in fattening ingredients like saturated and trans fats, added sugars, and sodium. Then, we highlight some of the foods you want to *start* eating instead—the recipes, products, and restaurant dishes that are lower in calories and other tummy-troubling ingredients and higher in belly-slimming, fat-releasing nutrients such as fiber, monounsaturated fatty acids, calcium, or vitamin C.

To decide which foods to include, I enlisted the help of my friend Mindy Hermann, a registered dietitian who understands the way busy people eat. Together with the health team at Reader's Digest, we went aisle by aisle through the supermarket, analyzing more than 40,000 products and prepared foods to pick out those that would be easiest to find and prepare, friendliest to your waistline, and good for your whole body. Then we gathered information from popular chain restaurant menus, along with recipes for everyday dishes like pancakes, chili, spaghetti, meatloaf, and much more.

All the foods featured in Part Three can fit in one of the three meal plans and are marked accordingly. We've also listed calorie counts for each so that you can make substitutions more easily. You might notice that, in

"I want to be healthier and have more control over nutrition. I try to make smart choices, but with my work and travel schedule, often what's quick is not the best option." A busy executive here at Reader's Digest, Donna Lindskog, 47, knew what she needed to do to eat right. It's just that her busy work schedule got in the way. She'd lose track of what she ate, especially from the afternoon on, and tell herself that she'd do better tomorrow. But tomorrow was usually the same old story.

"I lost 12 pounds in 12 days!"

As a frequent business traveler and restaurant diner, Donna was shocked by the eye-popping calorie numbers on some menus. So she was glad to see the many options for eating on the road in the Stop & Drop meal plans. "I used to be afraid of being stuck in the airport terminal between business flights because of all of the tempting food choices. Now, I bring snacks with me and walk around the terminal instead of eating. I am in control."

Donna also changed her approach to eating in restaurants. "I ask more questions about how foods are prepared and am not afraid of making special requests. I used to think that ordering dressing on the side and dipping my fork in it wouldn't work, but I tried it and it really does."

Does it ever! Donna dropped 12 pounds in 12 days, despite taking two business trips during that time, and trimmed her waist by 5 inches.

Notwithstanding all her travels, Donna says that her biggest challenge is finding healthy meals when her husband and three kids order in foods like Chinese. But with a bit of sleuthing and planning, she can find things to eat so that she doesn't feel deprived.

"The plan is easy and offers lots of opportunities to either cook at home or eat on the go. I am hopeful, energized, and enthusiastic, and I look forward to continuing to lose the weight!"

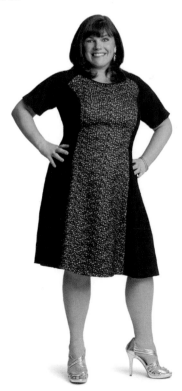

some cases, there doesn't appear to be a huge calorie difference between the foods we recommend you stop eating and those we suggest you should start eating. That's because calories are not the only factor that makes a food a smart and healthy choice. In making our recommendations, we also considered the amount and type of fat, sugar, sodium, and other nutrients in the foods and have highlighted those when they are significant. For the same reason, you may occasionally see that a Kickstart choice has more calories (but also more nutrition) than a Steady Loss or Maintain option.

How to Customize the Diet

How does the Stop & Drop Diet deliver on the promise of fast weight loss results? Primarily through the tried-and-true method of calorie restriction in its 1200-calorie Kickstart meal plan. For most people, 1200 calories is low enough that they'll lose up to a pound a day in the first week or so and high enough to provide the nutrition they need to fuel their body.

But what about the promise of maximum flexibility? As I noted earlier, what works for one person doesn't necessarily work for everyone. So we designed the Stop & Drop Diet to be easily customized for different lifestyles and tastes.

If you are the type of person who wants to be told what to eat from day to day, simply go to Chapter 5 and start picking out Kickstart meals to eat. (If even that is too loosey-goosey for you, then just pick the first choice of each meal on Day 1, the second choice on Day 2, etc.) Pick one breakfast, one lunch, one dinner, and one snack per day. After 1 week, go to Chapter 6 and start picking out Steady Loss meals—one breakfast, one lunch, one dinner, and up to two snacks per day. After 2 weeks, go to Chapter 7 and start picking out Maintain meals.

If you don't want to make huge changes to your lifestyle but just want to make smarter choices throughout the day, look up your favorite foods in Part Three to make sure that you are picking the versions with the fewest calories and most nutrition.

If you eat out a lot, pay particular attention to the restaurant dishes listed in Part Three (they come after the packaged foods in each category). A note: We've made our best efforts to ensure that the information is current, but because restaurants change their offerings frequently, you may find in a few cases that the choices we listed are no longer on the menu. When that happens, don't panic! If you can, visit the restaurant's website to find an alternate dish that has a similar number of calories. If you can't do that, ask your waiter to suggest something with a comparable number of calories.

Similarly, if you tend to rely on packaged foods for their convenience, pay particular attention to the packaged foods listed in Part Three. Again, we've made our best efforts to ensure that these are current, but food manufacturers, like restaurants, change their offerings (and their packaging) often. If you can't find one of the choices we've listed, look for a substitute with comparable foods and about the same number of calories.

If you like to cook, congratulations! You are most likely already consuming fewer calories than everyone else. But you can still trim further. You'll find some simple, five-ingredient recipes in Part Three, along with sidebars that highlight common ingredient choices and their respective calorie counts. If you're an experienced enough cook, you can make your own versions of any of the packaged and restaurant dishes; odds are, you'll come in lower in calories and higher in nutrition than they will.

Results in Real Life

To ensure that the plan was really as simple to follow, as flexible, and as effective as we wanted it to be, I recruited nine Reader's Digest readers and employees to try the plan with me. Every single one of us lost weight—at least a pound a day in the first 5 days for the majority of us. And everyone agreed that the plan was easy and convenient.

Angela Mastrantuono, 46, a construction accountant who lost 8 pounds in the first 5 days, raved, "It's so easy, you won't feel like you're on a diet."

Nora Healy, 52, a busy working mom here at Reader's Digest, was pleased that she and her family could eat similar foods—she didn't have to buy different foods or feel deprived. In addition, she reported, "The best feeling was finding meals I could eat while I was out on sales calls. Now I can go almost anywhere and find something healthy to eat."

A frequent restaurant-goer, Donna Lindskog, 47, loved the plan's "good choices, with easy, delicious meals."

And Karen Woytach, 33, our biggest loser, said, "The best part was the convenience of it all."

You'll see some of our testers' stories in Part One of the book, along with their tips and advice on how to make the diet work for you.

Part One
THE PROMISES

In creating the Stop & Drop Diet, I set out to deliver two things: (1) fast results—up to a pound of weight loss per day or even more—and (2) maximum flexibility to make this the easiest diet to follow. In Part One, I'll take you behind the scenes to show you how we constructed the diet to deliver on these promises and explain the science behind it.

Chapter 1
STOP BEFORE YOU DROP

Congratulations. You've decided you're ready to finally lose the weight. You've heard about some different approaches to weight loss and decided that this diet is the one for you. You're rarin' to go, and you want to start dropping the pounds *now*, right?

Well, hold on. I want to first ask you to STOP. What you've been doing to lose weight just hasn't worked, so you need to take the time to figure out why.

Maybe you are a serial dieter. Every time you hear about a new diet, you get excited and resolve that this will be it. You throw out all the food in your kitchen and buy all new products. Or you commit to cooking every meal every day for a whole month. You do great for a while. But then you go on vacation. Or you get busy at work. Or you just can't stand eating the same thing over and over again anymore. So you stop, and before you know it, you've regained the weight and then some.

Or maybe you've never really had a weight problem, but over the years you've noticed that you've had to loosen your belt a bit, and then a bit more. You keep thinking that it would be a good idea to lose a few pounds, but you hate the idea of having to follow a set meal plan. In fact, you hate the idea of having to plan your meals at all, and you definitely don't want to give up your wine/pizza/fill in the blank here with whatever your personal weakness is. (Cheese, glorious cheese, would be mine!)

In any case, you're clearly unhappy with your weight right now or you wouldn't have picked up this book. Before you dive into the plan itself, take a moment to stop and consider why you need to make some changes, what you need to stop doing, and how that can help you drop the pounds faster and keep them off.

Why Your Approach Isn't Working

You know that vegetables are good for you. You use skim milk in your coffee. On your sandwich, you opt for turkey over roast beef and whole wheat bread instead of white. So why does the number on the scale keep creeping up?

There could be a lot of reasons, of course, many of which have been the subject of successful diet books in their own right. You might be the victim of grain brain. Or maybe, especially if you're a woman over 40, it's your hormones. Perhaps, as I discussed in my last book *21-Day Tummy Diet*, you're suffering from an imbalance in your gut bacteria.

But even if you have one of these conditions, I bet there are a few, more basic reasons why you're not losing weight.

▶ Similar Foods Do Not Equal Similar Calories

Having written about health and weight loss for more than 20 years, I consider myself pretty savvy about food. But I was still surprised to find huge calorie differences between foods that look and sound very similar.

Take the humble burger, for instance. You've probably made your own patties for a backyard barbecue with some ground beef, topped with lettuce, tomato, and a couple of slices of cheese, all served on a regular hamburger bun. Squirt on some ketchup, and you've got a 570-calorie meal. That's not counting the fries or chips or anything else you might eat on the side.

Next time you grill, try making your patties with 95% lean ground beef. Replace the cheese with a half cup of sautéed onions or mushrooms, and use less ketchup. With just these few simple swaps, you've slashed 332 calories without sacrificing any taste.

I also got a wake-up call standing in front of the freezer case at the market. I picked up two different bags of vegetable-potato combos and expected their calories to be about the same. Imagine how surprised I was to see that 1 cup of the Alexia Harvest Sauté with Red Potatoes, Carrots, Green Beans and Onions had twice as many calories as the same portion of the Birds Eye Steamfresh Chef's Favorites Roasted Red Potatoes & Green Beans. The cause? An extra tablespoon of fat that I wouldn't have even tasted.

What about restaurant dishes? TGI Friday's has a couple of grilled steaks on the menu that sound very similar. But the 10-ounce Jack Daniel's Sirloin has 130 more calories than the 10-ounce Sirloin. Why? That special Jack Daniel's sauce has more carbs, most of which are probably sugar.

As tester Donna Lindskog discovered, it pays off to pay attention. "I learned to be more aware of the environment," she reported. "I also started asking more questions about the menu and how things were prepared, because I know sometimes you very naively say, 'I'll take the grilled chicken,' and meanwhile it's marinated in butter." (After just 5 days of paying attention and trimming her calories, Donna had dropped 6 pounds!)

Sneaky Calorie Culprits

How can such similar-sounding foods be so different in calories?
Fat and sugars.

FAT has more calories per gram than other nutrients, and it's easy to overdo. There's a reason why fat became demonized in the dieting world. Grab a bag of chips with your lunch or add a little extra oil or butter in cooking, and suddenly you've had 100 extra calories.

According to the U.S. government, our top sources of fat are desserts, pizza, cheese, chips, and salad dressing.[1] Plus, many types of fat—in particular, saturated and trans fats—can lead to serious health consequences if eaten in excess. A Harvard School of Public Health study back in 2006 concluded that for every 2 percent of calories that come from trans fats, heart disease risk goes up 23 percent.[2]

Of course, not all fats are bad for you—in fact, we all need some fat to survive. Some types of fat (MUFAs, anyone?) can even help us lose weight, as I outlined in my first book, *Flat Belly Diet!* But even the good fats need to be eaten in moderation. All too often, we simply eat too many of them because they're so concentrated in calories. Balance the fat in your diet so that you don't overshoot your calories for the day.

SUGARS Similarly, not all sugars are bad for us. Natural sugars, such as those found in fruit and dairy, are not a problem. But when food manufacturers started to mass-produce low-fat foods in the 1970s and '80s to appeal to dieters, they frequently pumped up the sugar to compensate for any loss in flavor. But sugars, of course, come with calories—lots of them—as well as their own negative health effects. Too much sugar has been implicated in many chronic health conditions. Chinese scientists found that drinking a lot of sugary beverages increased the chances of developing type 2 diabetes.[3] Researchers working on the decades-long Framingham Heart Study in Massachusetts observed a connection between drinking sugary beverages regularly and fatty liver disease, especially among people who are overweight or obese.[4]

And sugars are everywhere. They're not just in sodas, desserts, and candies. They're also in breads, salad dressings, pasta sauce, energy bars, and a lot of other foods that we don't think of as sweet. So of course we eat far too much of them—in fact, a whopping one out of every six calories we consume comes from one type of sugar or another.[5]

▶ Small Differences Add Up

Sometimes the differences between similar foods are not that dramatic. One slice of Pepperidge Farm Farmhouse Honey Wheat Bread is 120 calories. One slice of Pepperidge Farm Whole Grain Honey Wheat Bread is 110 calories. Will that 10-calorie difference pack on the pounds? Of course not. But go for a second slice of bread and spread both with butter (34 calories per teaspoon) rather than jam (19 calories per teaspoon), and now you've eaten an extra 50 calories.

That's still nothing that an extra minute or two on the treadmill can't handle, right? But on your lunch break, you run out to grab some soup. You like Au Bon Pain, so you duck in there to check out your choices. They have a Vegetarian Minestrone that you figure must be pretty healthy, and you're right. A small cup has just 80 calories, 1 gram of fat, and 4 grams of sugars—and it provides you with 3 grams each of filling fiber and protein. But you're hungry, so you opt for the larger bowl. And now you've eaten 80 extra calories. You've also eaten more sugars and fat.

For dinner, you're in the mood for pizza, so you pick up a frozen one. You figure that plain is better than pepperoni so you select the Freschetta Thin & Crispy 4 Cheese Medley Pizza. But it turns out that a serving of the Freschetta cheese pizza is actually 50 calories more than a serving of Newman's Own Thin & Crispy Uncured Pepperoni Pizza. You're trying to increase your vegetable intake, so you top it with green peppers and mushrooms. That adds another 12 calories.

For the day, you've eaten a total of 192 extra calories. Still not a big deal, really. But over time and in larger portions, these small differences do add up. Although experts are not sure of the exact number of calories in an extra pound of body fat, those 192 calories multiplied over 365 days equal 70,080 calories. At roughly 3500 calories per pound, you could add up to 20 pounds a year just by consistently adding these few extra calories.

Having said that, I want to emphasize that I do NOT want you to obsess over every last calorie. Therein lies madness! I was reminded of this while working on this book. We strive to be as accurate as possible in reporting calorie and nutrition information to you, so when Mindy first started collecting data on the tens of thousands of foods we considered including, she painstakingly recorded where she got the information—directly from the manufacturers' websites for brand-name packaged foods; from restaurant websites for specific restaurant dishes; and from reliable government databases for generic foods. By the time she passed the manuscript on to me to take a look, some of the information had already changed—manufacturers and restaurants had updated their sites and changed labels for some products. Then, when we started to collect foods to photograph, we discovered that some of the products were no longer being manufactured or offered at the restaurants. Our testers also found that some items touted as being available nationwide by the manufacturers and restaurants simply could not be found at their local grocery stores and chain locations.

As an author, it drove me crazy to have to keep updating information we'd already double- and triple-checked. As a dieter, it drove me even crazier. Because my husband's work schedule is more flexible than mine, he sweetly volunteered to shop for my first week on the Stop & Drop Diet. I picked out the meals that looked most appealing from the Kickstart meal plan, made up a shopping list, e-mailed it to him, and off he went. Then at work I started getting texts: "No Lean Cuisine Baked Chicken, Herb Roasted Chicken ok?" "Pepperidge Farm Whole Grain Honey Wheat or Farmhouse Honey Wheat Bread?" "What flavor Popcorners?"

At which point I realized both the enormity of the task I'd set for myself and the very great need for it. There's a lot of calorie and nutrition information out there, much of it contradictory and constantly changing. (If you happen to pick up the microwaveable bowl of Healthy Choice Tomato Basil Soup, for instance, it says one serving is 110 calories. But the Nutrition Facts label and the Healthy Choice website both say it's 130 calories!) Trying to keep up with it all would be a full-time job and then some. Since I already have a full-time job, there's no way I can keep recalculating my meal plans every time I need to make a substitution that has 20 more calories. The good news is that I don't need to, and neither do you.

As with most things in life, the best route is to take the middle ground. Pay attention to calories, because they do matter and they do add up. Use this book to help you identify the brand-name products and restaurant dishes that are the best choices, and follow the simple guidelines in Chapter 4 for picking substitutions when you can't find the ones we recommend. But don't fret if you end up with a dish that's a few calories more than the one we listed. Just write it down in your food journal and keep going with the rest of the diet. The key is simply to be aware of what you're eating and keep your calories in check over time.

▶ Portion Distortion

California Pizza Kitchen has a Chinese chicken salad with dressing I used to love—until I found out that it had 790 calories, 36 grams of fat, and 39 grams of sugars! Luckily, CPK offers half-size portions of its salads, so now I get a much more reasonable 395 calories, 18 grams of fat, and 19.5 grams of sugars. And no, I'm not hungry even though I'm eating only half as much; in fact, I don't even miss the extra. How can that be?

It turns out that my body never needed that much food at one sitting; I ate it just because it was there. Brian Wansink, PhD, director of the Cornell University Food and Brand Lab, pioneered research back in 2004 showing that the more food we are served, the more we eat. In a classic study published in 2005 in the *Journal of Nutrition Education and Behavior*, Dr. Wansink served a medium-size bucket of stale popcorn to some moviegoers and a large-size bucket to others. Guess who ate more popcorn? The people with the big bucket.[6]

Barbara Rolls, PhD, professor and chair of Nutritional Sciences at Penn State University, had similar results with potato chips, macaroni and cheese, and other foods. In one study, Dr. Rolls and her colleagues changed the size but not the price of a pasta entrée without telling their study subjects. People who bought the bigger portion—1½ times bigger—ate nearly 50 percent more calories from the pasta.[7] The same thing happened when she served some people bigger drinks: They drank more calories.[8]

Whether it's because we were told to "clean your plate" as kids or because we hate to waste food or we just don't notice how much we're eating, this tendency to eat all we're given has become a big problem. That's because the portions we're given have grown. Marion Nestle, PhD, a professor in the Department of Nutrition, Food Studies, and Public Health at New York University, and her colleague Lisa R. Young, PhD, RD, among others, have also found that beverages, fries, burgers, and muffins, to name just a few, have been getting bigger and bigger. Many are three or four times larger than the portions the government recommends! For example, in the mid-1950s, the only size fries sold by McDonald's matched the "small" size in 2001 and was one-third the size of a "large" order. Burger King sold only a 3.9-ounce burger in the 1950s; in 2002, the burger was more than three times that size.[9]

With our packages, plates, and portions so much bigger than they ought to be, it's no wonder that our calorie intake—and therefore our collective waistlines—are also so much bigger than they ought to be. If the only change you make to your eating habits is to make your portions smaller, you will shed calories. So remember when I told you not to obsess about counting calories? What you should obsess about instead is recalibrating your portions.

Yes, I know it's a pain to break out the measuring cups and food scale at every meal. If you've dieted in the past, you've probably done this exercise before, so you think you have a pretty good idea of what 3 ounces of ground beef or a half cup of rice looks like. But humor me and do it again, at least for the first few days. I did, and I was surprised to find that I routinely drank a quarter cup more milk and added a quarter cup more cereal than I thought to my morning meal. That added up to about 50 extra calories a day, or 18,000 over a year's time. And it turns out I'm not the only one who underestimates the portions I eat. In a study published in the *American Journal of Preventive Medicine*, researchers found that participants using a food diary underestimated their calorie intake by up to 17.7 percent compared to when they also wore a camera to record what they ate.[10]

That's why you'll see that we've specified not just what foods to eat in the meal plans in Part Two, but how much of each food. Similarly, in Part Three, we've listed the appropriate serving size for each food that we recommend you start eating. Pay attention to these numbers! In most cases, we've stuck to the serving sizes listed by the food manufacturers and to the portions served by the restaurants. But in some cases, we found that the calorie count for the recommended serving size was just too high to fit into our meal plans. Rather than forbidding that food entirely, you'll see that we sometimes recommend partial portions. If that feels wasteful to you, try sharing with some friends or saving some for a later meal.

When you are cooking for yourself, it's relatively easy to measure all your ingredients to make sure you're getting the right portions of everything. When you're eating packaged foods, read carefully! Sometimes the serving size will be easy to measure—1 whole package, 1 hot dog, ½ cup soup. Sometimes it won't—61 veggie straws, 23 chips, ⅐ package. We've tried to stick with portions that are easy to measure, but again sometimes the calorie counts for the obvious portions just don't work in our meal plans.

In restaurants, of course, it's a lot harder to know just how much food you're getting. You have no control over how much of each ingredient goes into each dish, what size plates your food will be served on, or how much food will be placed on your plate. So for restaurant foods, we've worked from nutrition information listed on each chain's website and calculated accordingly. As much as possible, to make it simple, we have chosen dishes where you can eat the whole thing. One big exception to this is in the Main Dishes section, where the default portion listed is the entrée only with no side dishes (even if they come with the entrée). We left off the side dishes to give you better control over total calories. Plus, many of the restaurants have healthier side dishes than the ones that are served with the dish. But because restaurant dishes in general tend to be much higher in calories than the recipes or the packaged food, we frequently suggest partial portions. If a restaurant offers a half-size or lunch portion or other sort of special portion on the menu, we often choose that instead and specify it. If not, you'll need to order the whole dish and just eat the portion specified.

Still unsure how much to eat in the restaurant? Check out our "Portion Guide" at right to help you right-size your portions and stick to the meals and foods as listed in Parts Two and Three.

Portion Guide

To make it easier to eat right-size portions when you're away from home, keep these basic portion size guidelines in mind:

1 teaspoon of butter or oil	=	The tip of your thumb
1 tablespoon of dressing	=	Half a shot glass
1 tablespoon of peanut butter or chopped nuts	=	Half a table tennis ball
1-ounce serving of cheese	=	Your whole thumb or a table tennis ball
1-ounce serving of pretzels or chips	=	One cupped handful
¼ cup croutons	=	A golf ball
1 cup chopped, sliced, or cubed fruit	=	A baseball
1 small pear, apple, or orange	=	A standard lightbulb
1 small banana	=	The length of your hand from the tip of your pointer finger to the base of your palm
1 medium pear, apple, or orange	=	A baseball
¾ cup cereal	=	A small coffee mug
1 small roll	=	The bulb portion of a lightbulb
1 medium potato	=	A computer mouse or a bar of soap
½ cup rice or pasta	=	The bulb portion of a lightbulb or half a baseball
3- to 4-ounce serving of meat, poultry, or fish	=	The palm of your hand (without fingers or thumb), a minipack of tissues, or a deck of cards
2 cups baby lettuce or spring greens	=	Two big fistfuls

What to Stop

Sneaky calorie culprits, small calorie differences, and ever-larger portions all add up to quite a bit of calorie creep. How do you stop extra calories in unhealthy versions of your favorite foods from sabotaging your weight loss? Dodge these top 10 diet pitfalls.

▶ Stop Eating When You're Not Hungry

Food is everywhere today. It's nearly impossible to go through even an hour without coming face-to-face with snack foods, candy, or other tempting treats in stores, at the gas station, on the desks of colleagues, and at the cash register of your favorite store. And what's the typical and predictable reaction? Eating, even if you're not hungry. Dr. Wansink dedicated a whole book to what he calls mindless eating—that is, eating for reasons other than being hungry.[11]

A lot of us are slaves to the clock. When I was growing up, my mother had dinner on the table promptly at six o'clock. Even if I wasn't especially hungry then, you can be sure I ate—and I cleaned my plate, because that's what we did in our house. Who knows how many extra calories I ate that way? I'm not saying that your meals should be unplanned. In fact, it's best to make sure you eat regularly to keep from getting so ravenous that you lose control and can't stop eating. But if you're in the habit of eating when the clock says to, instead of when you're actually hungry—which researchers at the University of Minnesota found is one of the main reasons people eat when they do[12]—you tend to lose touch with what "hungry" feels like and eat more than you really need.

So keep your schedule flexible if possible and listen to your tummy. On weekends, for example, I find that two main meals is all I need or want. I'll linger over coffee (or go for a run), then find it's 11, sometimes 12 o'clock before I'm hungry enough to want to eat. Or I'll have a healthy breakfast, then get caught up in my day and have what I call an "afternoon dinner" at 3 or 4.

Also, learn to stop eating when you're full. I still find myself automatically cleaning my plate, like I did as a kid, with no sense of when my hunger has really abated. And guess what? Members of the "Clean Plate Club" tend to have a heavier body weight, according to researchers in Liverpool, UK.[13]

I won't be going into a lot of detail on strategies in this book. But I encourage you to explore new habits that could help you get back in touch with your own feelings of hunger and fullness. You might want to write down what you eat and how you feel. For a lot of people, keeping a journal puts the brakes on their eating; writing down every bite brings them face-to-face with their food decisions. Another approach is to eat more slowly. Or to concentrate on tasting every bite. Each person is different, so create your own playbook! The most important thing is to stop before you start eating, so that you can go from being mindless about meals to being mindful.

▶ Stop Eating When You're Distracted

Do you see crumbs or smudges on your computer keyboard, the touch screen of your phone, or your TV's remote control? That's a telltale sign that you're doing other things while you're eating. Don't get me wrong. I'm all for multitasking, and I definitely have days when I eat in front of the computer. Here's the problem. Ask me how it tasted and I might not be able to tell you, because I was preoccupied by my work.

Have you ever grabbed a bag of chips or pretzels, sat down on the couch for your favorite show, and eaten the whole bag by the end of the show? Researchers in Ireland interviewed a group of 66 adults on what made portion control difficult. One of the main factors, they reported, were elements of the eating environment—socializing with friends and family, watching television, or working on a computer or phone—that diverted their attention away from what they were eating.[14] And a review of two dozen studies showed that being distracted at one meal may even cause people to eat more later in the day![15]

Again, mindful eating is key. Focus on what you're eating, and I bet you'll enjoy your food much more—and you'll also enjoy knowing that you haven't stuffed yourself with empty extra calories.

▶ Stop Eating Everything You're Served

The U.S. Department of Agriculture issues *Dietary Guidelines for Americans* every five years, updating it based on the latest science. The guidelines make recommendations about the amount of different types of foods and nutrients we should eat to manage weight and maintain health, based on a 2000-calorie day. In 2011, the USDA unveiled a new icon, MyPlate, to accompany the guidelines. This was intended to make it easier for people to see at a glance what kinds of food they should eat and how much of each.

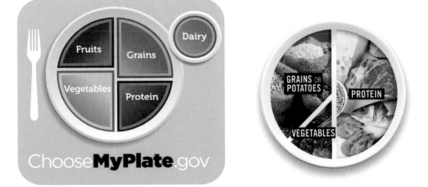

A dinner that follows the MyPlate recommendations would be approximately one-quarter protein, one-quarter grain, and half vegetable and fruit, plus a modest portion of dairy (such as a 16-ounce latte made with 1 cup each hot fat-free milk and coffee).[16] Now compare this to a typical restaurant dinner, especially at the better restaurants: about half protein, a big portion of grains or potatoes, and a vegetable garnish.

As you can see, the two dinners are nothing alike! With portions of some types of foods too big (usually meat, cheese, and grains) and portions of others too small (usually vegetables and fruits), the restaurant meal has too many calories and not enough nutrition. In fact, the government's data from "What We Eat in America" shows that the diets of restaurant eaters have more calories, protein, and carbs and less vitamin A, beta-carotene, and vitamin C—nutrients found mainly in fruits and vegetables.[17]

Unfortunately, this type of plate has become the norm. When we cook at home now, we portion out our meat, potatoes, and vegetables this way. Frozen dinners can be out of balance, too, with two carb-heavy side dishes and not much in the way of green veggies.

How do we stop blindly eating everything we're given? In the meals in Part Two, you'll see that in restaurant meals, Mindy frequently gives instructions for you to not eat certain things that are usually served with a given dish. Then, she often pairs the entrée with different sides. In the Kickstart meal plan, for instance, in Dinner #14, you'll order the Chili's Fajitas and eat one-third of the steak, peppers, onions, and toppings (salsa and jalapeños) in a single tortilla, with a side order of avocado added for its filling healthy fats. This helps to rebalance the nutrition as well as keep calories in check.

Similarly, with packaged foods, you'll see that you're not always eating the whole package and you're often pairing that with a salad or steamed vegetable, to keep the calorie level down while pumping up the nutrition. To keep it simple, I asked Mindy to keep the modifications reasonable. So we may ask you to eat half a package of something but (with a few exceptions) not one-seventh of a package.

"You realize that when you have a meal, you can eat on and on," noted tester Eileen Supran, 48, who dropped 4 pounds in 5 days. "[The Stop & Drop Diet] stopped me short . . . and I felt content." Angela Mastrantuono, 46, who dropped 8 pounds in 5 days, concurred: "I realized that I had been shoveling a lot of stuff in my mouth, not ending up full or satisfied, so I was always hungry. But with the meal plan, much less food ended up being more than enough."

Don't be afraid to ask for special accommodations at a restaurant. Even in fast-food chains, you can often order off the menu, as I discovered when I was traveling alone with my then 3-year-old daughters. McDonald's was the only place we could stop for breakfast, and at the time, they were picky about what they would eat. They asked for scrambled eggs, and I couldn't bear the idea of ordering two whole Big Breakfast plates, only to toss most of it (or worse, be tempted to finish off the sausages, hash browns, and biscuits myself). So I asked if I could just get two orders of the eggs that came with the Big Breakfast, and they were happy to oblige.

▶ Stop Dining Out for Every Meal

There are some restaurant meals that we all know we really shouldn't eat on a regular basis. During my annual reunion with my high school girlfriends, for instance, I won't hesitate to dig into a loaded burger *and* polish off a whole plate of fries, while also enjoying a cocktail—even though I know that's a meal that contains way more calories, fat, and sugar than I need.

But these occasional indulgences are not the problem. The problem is, we are eating out more and more often—over a 40-year period from 1970 to 2010, we nearly doubled the percentage of calories we get from food away from home.[18] And we are all too often unaware of how many calories are in the dishes we eat. A study of fast-food eaters in Philadelphia and Baltimore found that they underestimated their meal by up to 400 calories![19]

As I was researching this book, I ran across and saved a wonderful *New York Times* article called "What 2,000 Calories Looks Like."[20] It showed photos of 2000-calorie meals from popular chain restaurants—and you know what the scary thing is? They don't look like a lot of food at all. One photo that stands out in my mind shows a steak and a martini. No potatoes, no sides, no gravy; just the steak and cocktail add up to 2000 calories. That's more than the calories you should have in a whole day. Now that stopped me in my tracks!

I want to reassure you that I am not telling you to stop dining out. In fact, many of the foods, meals, and snacks in the book come from restaurant and fast-food menus because that's how we eat. It's part of our lifestyle.

But it's also one of the biggest calorie traps we face. Restaurant meals tend to be higher in calories, saturated fat, and sodium than homemade meals, and lower in calcium, fiber, and other weight-friendly nutrients. Consider, for instance, the Red Lobster Create Your Own Combination of Parrot Isle Jumbo Coconut Shrimp, Walt's Favorite Shrimp, and Shrimp Linguini Alfredo. Served with a Caesar salad, french fries, and a Cheddar Bay Biscuit, and washed down with a Traditional Lobsterita margarita, this seafood meal adds up to a whopping 3600 calories, with 37 grams of saturated fat and 7390 milligrams of sodium. No wonder it made the list of the 2015 Xtreme Eating Award's 9 Worst Chain Restaurant Meals of the Year, as identified by the Center for Science in the Public Interest.[21]

One of the kindest things we could do for our waists and our overall health would be to eat out less often. If you're in the habit of always grabbing a bagel on the way in to work, stock up instead on Nature's Own Plain Thin-Sliced Bagels. If you like a deli hoagie for lunch, bring your own turkey sub. You get the idea.

And when you do eat out, look for entrées that are grilled or baked, not fried or smothered in sauce, and for side dishes that pile on the veggies (again, you're looking for steamed, sautéed, or otherwise simply prepared vegetables). Any restaurant that is part of a chain with at least 20 outlets will soon be required to list calories and to have other nutrition information available.[22] This is making it easier for consumers like us to figure out what we're actually eating and to plan accordingly.

▶ Stop Picking Just the "Healthy" Brands

Common assumptions: Fast food is unhealthy, frozen dinners have too much sodium, and smoothies are the best way to lose weight. And if you're trying to drop pounds and be healthy, your best bet is to choose foods from the restaurants and brands that emphasize fresh, whole ingredients and prepackaged portions, like Chipotle, Jamba Juice, KIND, Lean Cuisine, and Weight Watchers. Right? That's what I thought before I started working on the Stop & Drop Diet.

Picking healthy foods is not as simple as finding a "healthy" brand and sticking to it. It's true that fresh, whole ingredients are better for you than processed and preserved foods. But there is such a thing as too much of a good thing. In a February 2015 *New York Times* article, a group of reporters gathered 3000 meal orders from Chipotle—which proudly proclaims on its website, "We're all about simple, fresh food without artificial flavors or fillers"[23]—and calculated the calories, saturated fat, and sodium in them. Guess what they found? The typical order, a burrito, weighed in at more than 1000 calories! It also had as much sodium as is recommended for an entire day, plus three-quarters of the recommended daily limit for artery-clogging saturated fat.[24]

This isn't to say, of course, that you can't find a healthy meal at Chipotle. The same article highlights several Chipotle meals that clock in at around 545 calories, including crispy steak tacos, a veggie bowl, and a carnitas burrito, and it's possible to get even lower by changing the fillings and toppings you choose.

KIND, another brand that touts itself as "healthy and tasty,"[25] was recently taken to task by the Food and Drug Administration, which found that several of its products did not meet the requirements to use the claims "good source of fiber," "no trans fats," "low sodium", "+ antioxidants," and "+ protein," among others.[26] In its defense, KIND noted on its blog, "Nuts, key ingredients in many of our snacks and one of the things that make fans love our bars, contain nutritious fats that exceed the amount allowed under the FDA's standard."[27] Having delved into the research on healthy fats for my first book, *Flat Belly Diet!*, I agree with KIND on this one.

That being said, the fact remains that many KIND bars *are* higher in calories or fat than, for instance, a Quaker or Nature Valley or Kashi bar. On the other hand, some Quaker, Nature Valley, and Kashi bars may be higher in calories and/or sugars and/or sodium than some KIND bars. The point is, every restaurant and every brand has some dishes and products that are healthier than others. In order to get the full story about any given food, you need to look beyond the brand and beyond the health claims spouted in advertisements and printed on the front of the box.

To make matters even more confusing, package claims can be misleading. David Benton, a professor in the Department of Psychology at Swansea University, Wales, gathered evidence about incorrect assumptions people make: that low-fat foods are lower in calories, low-cholesterol foods are low in fat, and organic foods have fewer calories.[28] Just as problematic, Dr. Wansink and researcher Pierre Chandon, also of Cornell University, found that people ate more M&Ms, and more calories, when the package said the M&Ms were low in fat.[29]

Finally, some good news! In collecting the data for this book, I was pleasantly surprised to find many smaller portion, lower-calorie, lower-fat options at fast-food restaurants—quite a bit more, in fact, than at most sit-down restaurants. A recent study by Ruopeng An, PhD, assistant professor in the Department of Kinesiology and Community Health at the University of Illinois at Urbana-Champaign, found that diners consume no more calories—but get more salt and cholesterol—at sit-down restaurants than at fast-food restaurants.[30] I was also happy to see that many packaged foods had a good balance of nutrients, especially calorie- and portion-sensitive brands like Weight Watchers Smart Ones, Lean Cuisine, and Healthy Choice.

▶ Stop Starving Yourself

At one of my first jobs, I had a co-worker who was a serial dieter. Every few months, she would announce that she was starting a new diet and warned us that she would be irritable because she would be so hungry. And she was. She would snap at anyone who reminded her about a deadline, she would grumble loudly that she couldn't join any office birthday parties, and she would constantly complain about how she was starving! And in the 3 years that I worked with her, she did not lose weight.

While it's true that in order to lose weight, you need to eat less, that does not mean you need to starve yourself! In fact, starving yourself often has the opposite effect. To your body, your extra fat is a necessary hedge against the day that there's no food to be had. We humans evolved during a time when there were no grocery stores or restaurants or even farms. How did our ancestors survive when there was a drought that killed off the leaves and berries they foraged? Or when they failed in the hunt? They lived off the fat they had built up during more plentiful times.[31] Which is why, when you suddenly slash the amount of food you're eating, your body reacts by hanging on to every bit of fat it can.[32]

The same thing happens when you skip meals. Skip breakfast and you're likely to overdo it at lunch since you're so hungry. Skip lunch and you may be too ravenous by dinner to make smart food choices. A study of eight years of data from the National Health and Nutrition Examination Survey (NHANES) showed that people who skip breakfast tend to be heavier and have a larger waist than those who eat a healthy breakfast.[33]

The conventional wisdom among the U.S. Department of Agriculture, National Institutes of Health, and many others is that in order to avoid this, you want to make gradual changes to your diet and lose weight slowly, about a pound or two a week. But while I'd certainly rather lose a pound or two than gain a pound or two a week, when I've set my mind to lose weight, that seems impossibly slow. That's why Mindy and I designed the Stop & Drop Diet in phases. The Kickstart phase lowers your calorie level enough that you'll drop the pounds fast at first. But then, to avoid the plateaus that come when your body gets used to the lower calorie levels, you'll switch to the higher-calorie Steady Loss phase. An article published in *Lancet* recommends just this type of "step change" to maximize weight loss over time.[34] And while you may be hungry at first on the Kickstart phase, I promise you won't starve. Mindy made sure that the meals in every phase generally have a good balance of nutrition to satisfy your body and keep it fueled healthfully.

▶ Stop Forbidding Foods

The Atkins Diet. The South Beach Diet. The Paleo Diet. The Dukan Diet. So many popular diets today recommend cutting out or drastically cutting down on carbohydrates that there must be something to the low-carb thing, right? Well, it's true that, on average, Americans eat more carbs than we really need, especially refined carbohydrates like those in white bread, pasta, cakes, and cookies. Among our top sources of calories, in fact, are cakes and cookies, breads, pizza, pasta, and sugary drinks.[35] So if you cut back on these foods, you will automatically slash your calorie consumption and lose weight. And, because excess consumption of refined carbs has been associated with diabetes, heart disease, and a host of other chronic diseases, you'll be healthier if you eat fewer of them.

But of course, when you suddenly stop eating an entire food group, you are automatically cutting calories and your body reacts accordingly. It

Party planner Diane Rohan personifies nonstop movement. She takes Zumba classes 5 days a week at a studio near her home, supplements her classes by using a stairclimber, does 50 sit-ups a day, and still finds time to walk and care for foster puppies. That's why she was so frustrated that her weight had gotten stuck. "Between my slow thyroid and now menopause, I can't seem to lose weight with regular methods of cutting calories and exercising," she complained before she started the Stop & Drop Diet. "A couple of years ago, I lost 10 pounds that I want to keep off, plus I want to lose 20 pounds more."

"I am a foodie, and I love to cook."

A veteran dieter, Diane noted, "The eating plan made me more conscious of what I'm doing. I knew what to do but didn't do it before this plan. When I go to a restaurant now, I don't eat a three-course meal. My husband and I might have appetizers and share an entrée instead."

Diane worked hard to stay on track and make the most of any menu and meal. Faced with a restaurant menu limited to fried, cheesy, oily, or salty foods, she took only small portions. She was tempted by a Wendy's burger—a few Wendy's meals are listed in our swaps—but as an avid cook, she decided instead to Google the ingredients and calories and make her own version. She maintained her morning latte routine, using half of her breakfast milk for her cereal and the other half for her coffee drink. She also found that eating every 4 hours or so made a big difference for her.

After just 5 days, Diane had shed 7 pounds. After 3 weeks, she was thrilled to find that jeans and pants she couldn't zip were now back in her wardrobe. "My first 3 weeks were rough because I was sick, had puppies to care for, and didn't go outside much because it was so cold. The odds were stacked against me, but I kept at it. I look forward to continuing my meal plan and workouts and moving closer to my weight goal."

thinks you're starving and responds by slowing your metabolism and hanging on to every calorie it can.[36] Plus, your body misses the nutrients it's not getting. For example, dairy products are a top source of calcium, vitamin D, and potassium. Eliminate them and you'll have to work hard to make up those nutrients. There's a psychological aspect to it, too. Tell me I can't have something or restrict the amount I can eat, and suddenly it's the only thing I want.[37] Next thing you know, you're craving those forbidden foods like nobody's business, and you feel like you'd mow down your own mother to get to a piece of bread.

The same is true for low-fat diets, low-salt diets, and pretty much any other diet that forbids specific foods. Which is not to say that these types of diets can't be healthy. But most people find that they're hard to sustain over time because they often require a lot of cooking or buying specialty food items. And a diet certainly won't work if you don't follow it.

We made the Stop & Drop Diet as flexible and easy to follow as we could. And we made it healthy. As you'll see when we talk about the nutritional parameters we followed for the meals, the Stop & Drop Diet is relatively low in fat, carbs, and salt. It can easily be made vegetarian or vegan, if that's what you prefer. But it doesn't forbid any foods. Because let's face it, we know you're going to eat cake sometimes. After all, what's the point of living if you can't enjoy yourself? We're just going to show you what kind of cake and how much you can eat so you can still enjoy weight loss.

▶ Stop Relying on Dieting Alone

I've told this story in other books, but I think it bears repeating. When I was in my thirties, I worked at *Fitness* magazine and, knowing all the research about the health benefits of exercise, I was inspired to work out a dozen hours a week. Because I exercised so much, I figured that I didn't really need to pay too much attention to how much I ate, especially since I stuck to mostly healthy foods—fruits, vegetables, whole grains, lean proteins, and fat-free dairy. But by the time my forties rolled around, I found myself about 10 pounds heavier than I wanted to be.

Because I hated the idea of limiting what I ate, I tried to lose the weight by exercising even more. I added another half hour to my daily walks and stepped up the tempo. I tried a new dance class. I also started strength-training to increase my muscle mass and boost my metabolism. But after three months, I'd only lost a measly pound and a half.

Clearly, relying on exercise alone was not enough to lose weight. Diet is key. But the converse is also true. While you *can* lose weight even if the only movement you make all day is walking from your bed to your desk chair, it's much easier and faster to drop pounds if you combine diet and exercise. If you are burning an extra 200 to 300 calories per day, that's 200 to 300 calories less you have to carve out from your diet to get the same calorie deficit. Plus, exercise generates natural endorphins, so you feel better and have more energy even if you are a little hungry. All of which makes it easier to stick with the diet.

And once you've lost the weight, exercise has also proven to be key to keeping it off. According to the National Weight Control Registry, established in 1994 to identify and investigate the characteristics of people who have successfully lost weight and kept it off for more than a year, 94 percent increased their physical activity in order to lose weight, with the most frequently reported form of exercise being walking. To keep it off, 90 percent report that they exercise an average of an hour a day.[38]

That's why exercise is an integral part of the Stop & Drop Diet. I won't spend a lot of time talking about exercise in this book because, frankly, fitness is much less complicated than food. In all three phases of the diet—and indeed, for the rest of your life—just walk an hour a day, every day. If you are doing other types of exercise, great. If you can do more than an hour a day, great. But at a minimum, move at least an hour a day, and your body will reward you. Remember that you can break this up into smaller chunks. You can do it wherever you are. Walk the dog in the morning, walk around the block at lunchtime, walk down the hallway to talk to a colleague, walk around the grocery store buying your Stop & Drop foods—you get the idea.

Our testers didn't let a bitterly cold winter stop them from walking! Nora Healy reported one day that "I ended up getting my one hour of walking to and from the train because our cars were under 3-foot snowdrifts!" Karen Woytach got her hour vigorously playing in the snow going up and down hills with sleds, while Randi Zelkin took her workout indoors, noting, "I've been walking around my house in circles for a while now, and my husband thinks I'm nuts!"

▶ Stop Thinking It's All or Nothing

Recently, while working on a particularly tough deadline, I didn't have a chance to pack my usual greens and protein for lunch. Instead, I gratefully grabbed a couple slices of pizza that were left over from another department's office party. I detoured by the candy bowl in the art department a few times during the afternoon. That night, after taco dinner with the family (it's the twins' favorite!), I took out my cute ice-cream sundae cup, scooped out a quarter cup of vanilla frozen yogurt, sank into my favorite big armchair, and savored it. Usually I'm satisfied with that, especially if I get caught up in a good book and don't want to get up again to get more. But this time, I went back to the freezer and scooped out another quarter cup. When I looked in the carton, though, I thought, "Oh, there's not much left, I might as well finish it."

Sound familiar? If you have a day like this every so often and get right back on track, it's no big deal. The danger comes when you think, "I've blown my diet already, I might as well have that extra piece of cake." Losing weight is not an all-or-nothing proposition. If you have a 2400-calorie day like I did that day, but then go right back to a 1200-calorie Kickstart day or even a 1600-calorie Steady Loss day, you will still lose weight. But if you have another 2400-calorie day and then another, you will plateau, then start to gain back the weight.

To avoid these dire consequences, just keep coming back to your Kickstart and Steady Loss meals anytime you overdo it. The beauty of the Stop & Drop Diet is that it is designed to be flexible and nothing is forbidden. So it's tough to totally "blow it" and really easy to get back on track even if you do.

▶ Stop Feeling Bad about Your Weight

If you get depressed every time you step on a scale, or only see your fat butt when you look in the mirror, or refuse to have a photo taken because you're ashamed of what you look like, then you need to stop. Because I'll tell you a secret: No matter what you weigh, if you don't love your body, you will never truly win the weight loss battle. If you feel guilty about your eating habits and ashamed of your body, you will always feel deprived. While you may lose weight initially on the diet, you will soon slide back to your old food choices and gain it all back again.

The only way to finally, truly lose the weight and keep it off for good is to stop feeling bad about your weight and your body. If you love and respect your body, it will not feel like a chore to research restaurant entrees before you go out to eat or to read nutrition labels in the grocery store or to cook for yourself and your family. Instead, it will be a privilege to take care of yourself by making smart, healthy food choices.

Focus on how much better you feel physically and mentally. One study showed that people who reported feeling alive and energetic were more motivated and more successful at maintaining their weight loss.[39] Our testers all reported feeling more energetic and more self-confident on the diet, too. Nora Healy noted, "My daughter and I went to Nordstrom Rack, and I just felt so much better about everything I was putting on. I tried on different clothes, and I feel more youthful. I have a bigger spring in my step."

What to Start

When you stop before you eat, you have time to:

▶ **CHECK IN WITH YOUR BODY.** Before you take a bite, ask yourself if you're actually hungry or if you're eating out of boredom, stress, or just habit.

▶ **READ LABELS.** The most important number for weight loss is, of course, the calories per serving. But you'll also want to look at a few key nutrition facts, in particular fat, sugars, and sodium, to make sure that you don't take in too many of these fattening ingredients. One study showed that label readers weighed less![40]

▶ **MEASURE YOUR FOOD.** As I noted before, portions are important, and all too many of us have lost sight of how much food we should be eating. So invest in a food scale and keep a measuring cup and spoons handy.

▶ **GIVE THANKS.** For your hardworking body, with all its imperfections. For the food on your table. For the chance to get to your healthy weight.

▶ **MAKE SMART CHOICES.** Part Two will teach you how to put together nutritionally balanced meals anywhere you go. Part Three will show you how to avoid unhealthy versions and instead choose the best options for everything from breakfast pastries to pasta to ice creams and other frozen desserts.

These are the keys to finally losing weight and keeping it off. Even if you haven't been successful in the past, you *can* lose weight on the Stop & Drop Diet. First, the eating plan is fast and easy. Our testers' results prove it! Everyone lost weight, and they all loved not having to think hard about their meals. Second, you control your diet. With three different calorie levels, you can choose how much you cut and how fast you lose. In the next chapter, I'll show you how.

Chapter 2
CAN YOU REALLY DROP A POUND A DAY?

I bet you've heard that the rule of thumb for safe, effective, and lasting weight loss is a gradual approach, in which you lose a pound or two a week. But I know from personal experience—and I've heard from thousands of readers—that when you start a diet, you really just want to lose weight fast. And that if you don't, you get bored and discouraged and start to cheat. Besides giving you a great psychological boost right out of the gate, a breakthrough study says that losing weight quickly may also help you keep it off longer.

When researchers from the University of Florida analyzed data on 262 middle-age women who were struggling with obesity, they found that the women who had initially dropped weight most quickly tended to shed more weight overall and maintain the weight loss longer than those who had a more gradual start. In the year after the 6-month intervention phase, just 16.9 percent of women in the slow weight-loss group had reached the goal of shedding 10 percent of their overall body weight. In contrast, 35.6 percent of participants in the moderate weight-loss group and 50.7 percent in the fast group reached their goal.[41] Similarly, a European review of multiple weight management programs found that people who lost weight quickly found it easier to keep it off.[42]

That being said, plenty of crash diets, supplements, cleanses, and detoxes out there do strip off the pounds . . . but also strip you of energy, health, and enjoyment. That's not healthy, it's not sustainable, and it's certainly no fun.

That's why I asked registered dietitian Mindy Hermann to construct an eating plan that delivers fast results while still supplying all the essential nutrients you need. The Stop & Drop Diet is healthy, balanced, and gives you energy to spare. And it helped our testers drop a pound a day or even more: Karen Woytach, 33, a busy mom of three young kids, shed 10 pounds in just 5 days and 13½ pounds in 12 days! Diane Rohan, 51, lost 7 pounds in 5 days even though she was battling the hormonal fluctuations of menopause, which usually slows weight loss. And Donna Lindskog, 47, dropped 6 pounds in 5 days and 12 pounds in 12 days, despite a busy travel schedule. Now let's learn how you can do the same.

Can I Really Drop a Pound a Day without Starving?

As every dieter knows, weight loss is governed by a simple equation: Calories consumed – calories burned = pounds lost.

But, as every dieter also knows, living by this equation is hard to do. First of all, it can be difficult to figure out just how many calories *you* need to drop in order to lose weight because that number is different for each person. Second, it can be tough to assess how many calories you've actually consumed (and burned) unless you measure everything down to the teaspoon or limit yourself to packaged foods with calorie labels. Finally, it turns out that the equation is not completely accurate, after all. Losing weight is not all about the calories. Certain nutrients help you lose weight, without reducing your calorie intake. Others can sabotage your weight loss efforts, even if they don't add calories.

Luckily, the Stop & Drop Diet takes all of this into account, so you don't need to count calories, fat or sugar grams, or anything else. You just need to stop eating unhealthy versions of your favorite foods, start eating what we suggest instead, and enjoy our delicious meals to drop the pounds.

▶ Drop Calories

How many calories do you need to cut in order to lose a pound? It depends on a lot of different factors—your gender, your age, and your starting weight, not to mention what you typically eat, the amount of sodium in your diet, how much you exercise, and how recently you tried to lose weight.

The general rule of thumb that's been used for years by scientists is that a deficit of 3500 calories will lead to a pound of fat loss. David Allison, PhD, a professor at the University of Alabama, questions this premise because not every person loses a pound by cutting 3500 calories.[43] Researchers are trying to tease out the reasons why some people lose quickly and some don't, why some people keep on losing weight and some don't. In the meantime, I am as frustrated as you are that science doesn't really have an answer to what seems like a simple question.

Still, for most Americans of average weight and height, the 3500-calorie deficit is a good place to start. If you can cut 3500 calories out of your day, you will lose weight and quickly. In order to cut that many calories and still have enough to eat, you'd have to be eating almost 5000 calories a day—about 2.5 times the average calorie intake used by the USDA on food labels. I couldn't believe some Americans actually eat that much. But consider the following example:

STOP EATING		START EATING	
BREAKFAST—Dunkin' Donuts		**BREAKFAST—Dunkin' Donuts**	
Bacon, Egg, and Cheese on a Biscuit	470 calories	Bacon, Egg, and Cheese on an English muffin	290 calories
Medium Caramel Latte with regular milk	350 calories	Small Caramel Coffee with regular milk	35 calories
TOTAL	**820 calories**	**TOTAL**	**325 calories**
LUNCH—Chipotle		**LUNCH—Chipotle**	
Burrito with chicken, white rice, beans, fajita veggies, corn salsa, guacamole, sour cream, cheese, and lettuce, plus a side of chips and salsa	1940 calories	Burrito bowl with chicken, black beans, fajita veggies, tomato salsa	340 calories
TOTAL	**1940 calories**	**TOTAL**	**340 calories**
DINNER—TGI Friday's		**DINNER—TGI Friday's**	
Rib-Eye Steak with Langostino Lobster Topping	820 calories	½ of a 6 oz Sirloin	165 calories
House Salad, bleu cheese dressing, breadstick	420 calories	House Salad, vinegar, breadstick	210 calories
Sweet Potato Fries	390 calories	½ order mashed potatoes	105 calories
½ of a Brownie Obsession	600 calories	Red wine (5 oz)	125 calories
Red wine (8 oz)	200 calories		
TOTAL	**2430 calories**	**TOTAL**	**605 calories**
DAY TOTAL 5190 calories		**DAY TOTAL 1270 calories**	

DROP: 3920 calories

Doesn't look like an unreasonable amount of food in that first column, does it? There's not even a snack or a drink with lunch! And you're eating only half of a brownie for dessert. But, as you saw in Chapter 1, restaurant meals are notoriously high in calories and other fattening ingredients. That's why we encourage you to stop dining out for every meal.

But eating at home doesn't automatically mean you'll eat fewer calories. Consider this example:

STOP EATING		START EATING	
BREAKFAST—Home		BREAKFAST—Home	
3 scrambled eggs with 1 slice cheddar cheese	387 calories	2 scrambled eggs with 1 Tbsp grated cheddar cheese	210 calories
Thomas' Honey Wheat Bagel with 2 Tbsp cream cheese	349 calories	Thomas' 100% Whole Wheat Bagel Thin with 1 Tbsp low-fat cream cheese	140 calories
Coffee with 2 Tbsp half-and-half	39 calories	Coffee with 2 Tbsp fat-free milk	10 calories
TOTAL	**775 calories**	**TOTAL**	**360 calories**
LUNCH—Home		LUNCH—Home	
Hamburger made with 8 oz 80% lean ground beef, on a kaiser roll with 2 Tbsp mayo	981 calories	Hamburger made with 4 oz ground turkey breast, on a whole wheat bun with 1 Tbsp ketchup	160 calories
6 oz Ore-Ida Extra Crispy Easy Golden Fries	380 calories	3 oz Ore-Ida Steak Fries	110 calories
1 cup deli coleslaw	540 calories	1 cup Dole Classic Coleslaw drizzled with vinegar, noncaloric sweetener to taste	20 calories
TOTAL	**1901 calories**	**TOTAL**	**290 calories**
SNACK—Home		SNACK—Home	
1 cup Haagen-Dazs Vanilla Bean ice cream	540 calories	½ cup Breyers Natural Vanilla ice cream	130 calories
TOTAL	**540 calories**	**TOTAL**	**130 calories**
DINNER—Home		DINNER—Home	
Stouffer's Classics Chicken Fettuccini Alfredo	570 calories	Weight Watchers Smart Ones Fettuccini Alfredo	250 calories
1 2¼-inch piece (⅙ package) Pepperidge Farm Five Cheese Garlic Bread	200 calories	1 cup salad with lettuce, tomatoes, cucumber, 4 sprays of olive oil, and vinegar	30 calories
½ cup (½ of a 9-oz package) Stouffer's Creamed Spinach	200 calories	½ cup (½ package) Birds Eye Creamed Spinach	90 calories
1 slice (⅙ pie) Sara Lee Oven Fresh Blueberry Pie	350 calories	½ cup blueberries	42 calories
TOTAL	**1320 calories**	**TOTAL**	**412 calories**
SNACK—Home		SNACK—Home	
6 oz Kim & Scott's Grilled Cheese Pretzel	480 calories	2 sticks Super Pretzel Pretzelfils Mozzarella	130 calories
2 12-oz bottles Sam Adams Double Bock	480 calories	1 12-oz bottle Amstel Light beer	95 calories
TOTAL	**960 calories**	**TOTAL**	**225 calories**
DAY TOTAL 5496 calories		**DAY TOTAL 1417 calories**	

DROP: 4079 calories

You'll see that in this example, on the "good" day, you're eating well over the 1200 calories you get on the Kickstart phase of the Stop & Drop Diet. If you wanted to cut back further on your calories, you could enjoy three full meals plus a treat and just drop one of the snacks.

But, you think, these examples don't reflect how you eat because you generally eat pretty healthfully—you go meatless at least once a week. So do many Americans. Today, vegetarian dishes are much easier to find on restaurant menus and in the market. And plenty of research studies show that people who eat a vegetarian diet are healthier. They weigh less and are less likely to get heart disease or diabetes. But guess what? It's possible for even a vegetarian day to add up to more than 5000 calories. Consider the example to the right.

I could go on, but I think you get the idea. Whether you eat out or eat in, cook or rely on packaged foods, or even go meatless, it's altogether too easy to eat more than 5000 calories a day—and altogether too many of us do. That's the bad news. The good news is, it's just as easy to cut 3500 calories out of your day. And, as you can see from these examples, you can do so while still eating a lot of the same kinds of foods (burgers, pancakes, pasta with cream sauce, even cheesecake).

▶ Eat Calories

So what's the magic calorie number? As I said, it depends on a lot of different factors. If you consult with a nutritionist or fitness trainer, or go online to search for the answer, you'll find a lot of complicated formulas that ask you to input your age, your gender, your height, your weight, your current calorie intake, how many hours a day you're active and at what intensity level, and on and on. If you do enough of these, you'll find that most of them give you about the same answer. It's no coincidence. Most of them first calculate your basal metabolic rate, the amount of calories your body burns when at rest—this is really the minimum number of calories you should eat. Then they add on some calories depending on your daily activity level (the more active you are, the more calories you get). This is what gives you the energy to get out of bed and do what you need to do.

(One of the more sophisticated versions is the Body Weight Simulator created by Kevin D. Hall, PhD, of the National Institute of Diabetes and Digestive and Kidney Diseases, as part of a research project attempting to more accurately predict weight loss in real life. You can try it for yourself here: http://www.niddk.nih.gov/research-funding/at-niddk/labs-branches/LBM/integrative-physiology-section/body-weight-simulator/Pages/body-weight-simulator.aspx.)

STOP EATING		START EATING	
BREAKFAST—Home		**BREAKFAST—Home**	
3 pancakes made from Bisquick Complete Simply Buttermilk with Whole Grain Pancake and Waffle Mix, topped with 1 Tbsp butter, 2 Tbsp maple syrup	**410 calories**	2 Van's 8 Whole Grains Pancakes	**160 calories**
		Chobani Fruit on the Bottom Strawberry Banana Greek Yogurt	**150 calories**
1 cup smoothie made with fruit and canned coconut milk	**674 calories**	½ cup sliced strawberries	**27 calories**
TOTAL	**1084 calories**	**TOTAL**	**337 calories**
SNACK—Home		**SNACK—Home**	
½ cup Planters Nut-rition Energy Mix	**380 calories**	2 Tbsp Planters Fruit & Nut Trail Mix	**80 calories**
TOTAL	**380 calories**	**TOTAL**	**80 calories**
LUNCH—Home		**LUNCH—Home**	
½ cup deli roasted vegetables and 2 slices provolone cheese on 4 oz focaccia bread	**508 calories**	2 Tbsp chopped marinated artichoke hearts, 2 slices roasted red peppers, ¼ cup arugula, 1 slice provolone cheese on 2 slices Pepperidge Farm Whole Grain Honey Wheat Bread	**315 calories**
1 cup Pacific Organic Hearty Tomato Bisque	**150 calories**	1 cup Imagine Organic Creamy Tomato Soup	**80 calories**
1 piece deli chocolate chip coffee cake	**800 calories**	1 cup fruit salad	**90 calories**
TOTAL	**1458 calories**	**TOTAL**	**485 calories**
DINNER—Cheesecake Factory		**DINNER—Cheesecake Factory**	
Four Cheese Pasta	**1240 calories**	Vegetable Chopped Salad	**280 calories**
Small Tomato & Mozzarella Salad	**490 calories**	¼ slice Original Cheesecake	**177 calories**
½ slice Original Cheesecake	**355 calories**		
TOTAL	**2085 calories**	**TOTAL**	**457 calories**
DAY TOTAL 5007 calories		**DAY TOTAL 1359 calories**	

DROP: 3648 calories

For most adult women of average height, size, and activity level, this works out to between 1200 and 1600 calories; for most adult men, to between 1500 and 2000 calories. That's why we chose these as the calorie levels for the three phases of the Stop & Drop Diet. Unless you are morbidly obese or a professional athlete, you should be able to get all the nutrition and energy you need from one of these three phases. If you do fall into one of those categories, or have any other health concerns, please consult with your doctor before starting this or any weight loss program. In Part Two, I'll give you a little more guidance about when to do which phase of the diet.

How do you ensure that you're getting only the calories you need and no more? Just follow the Stop & Drop meal plan! Mindy has carefully selected the best foods and dishes from the thousands of supermarket products and restaurant meals out there, measured out the correct portions, and calculated the calories (along with all the nutrition) so that you don't have to.

And, as you'll see when you flip to the meals and foods in Parts Two and Three, you don't have to restrict yourself to raw kale and quinoa to make up your 1200–2000 calories. While I've read the research about how preservatives and other additives in many processed foods can negatively impact your weight and your health—and I'm a big fan of clean eating and the whole foods movement (nothing tastes better than a juicy tomato plucked straight out of my own garden!)—I'm also a realist. As a busy working mom, I simply don't have the time to make pasta sauce from scratch or bake my own bread. If you do, more power to you! But if you don't, or if you can't because you hit a busy patch or have to travel, this book can help you pick the best options from packaged and restaurant foods. Are English muffins better than whole wheat toast? Is the Burger King grilled chicken sandwich lower in calories than the one from Wendy's? Can you ever enjoy a chocolate cake? These and many more questions are ones the Stop & Drop Diet will answer.

Nora Healy raved, "I felt like I discovered a lot of foods that were great, like the Good Food Made Simple Steel Cut Oatmeal. I'd never heard of the brand, but it was right there at Target." Said Angela Mastrantuono, "I have a friend who's the pickiest eater. And I told her this diet was made for her. I said, 'You can go to McDonald's and get a parfait, or you can go to Wendy's and get a burger.' This is for the everyday person."

▶ Burn Calories

So far we've only talked about the consumption side of the calorie equation, but of course you can and should burn calories, too. Want to lose weight even faster? Or want to enjoy a snack or dessert while still dropping

For Karen Woytach, 33, life changed with the birth of her third child and a subsequent job loss, turning her into a stay-at-home mom for the first time. Karen became a snacker, grabbing food when she had a free moment during her baby's naps rather than because she was hungry. The busy schedules of her two older children meant little time to exercise and lots of time spent in the car. Karen's goal is to do more activities with all three of her children and not be embarrassed about being too big to participate.

"I went down a whole dress size!"

"I came to Reader's Digest looking for a program that fits into my mom lifestyle. It had to allow me to pick foods I actually like to eat without keeping track of calories. And I have to be able to feed my family, too. If I have parameters I can work with and can feel good about the food I am eating, I am more likely to be successful."

Karen lost 10 pounds in the first 5 days of the plan, and went on to lose 20 in 4 weeks. She was thrilled to find plenty of meals that she really liked. "I LOVED the salads, and they are big enough to make me feel like I am eating a lot. I also followed the suggestion to break up meals into minimeals. Doing that really helped calm my hunger.

"This feels really good. After the first couple of days, I got into a groove. I changed my eating habits and learned how to balance my calories with healthy options. The plan didn't hit me over the head with scary lifestyle changes, and it was easy to integrate into feeding my family.

"I have energy and confidence now. I did a little clothes shopping for the first time since my daughter was born a year ago. Not only did I get a few great pieces of clothing, I went down a clothing size!! I can't wait to return to the body that my husband married."

pounds? Move more to burn more calories. If you already have a regular exercise routine, by all means keep it up (or, for even better results, change it up by taking a new class or trying new machines or routines).

But whether or not you already exercise, add a walk. Then make that walk a little faster and a little longer, until you are walking an hour a day. It's that easy. An hour a day may sound like a lot, but I promise it's doable. Remember that you don't have to do it all at once, and you don't need to do it at the gym. March in front of your TV for 15 minutes while you're watching the morning news, pace for 10 minutes in your office while you're on a conference call, power walk for 20 minutes during your lunch break, walk around the parking lot for 15 minutes while you're waiting to pick up the kids—and you're done. I personally strength-train twice a week and run twice a week, and I walk an average of 90 minutes a day on top of that.

As I mentioned before, our testers were able to get in their walking even under challenging circumstances, and they all felt better when they did. "I feel like I'm healthier because I'm incorporating more than the amount of exercise I was doing before," said Diane Rohan. "I'm super happy." Donna Lindskog noted, "Even at the airport, instead of sitting at the terminal, I walked around the terminal just to get some movement, and I felt good."

Again, the amount of weight you lose by walking will vary depending on your weight, your general fitness level, your walking speed, and many other factors, but you can burn up to 350 calories in an hour of brisk walking.[44] Plus, you'll feel better and help to ward off heart disease, type 2 diabetes, and a host of other health issues. If you can, grab some friends to walk with you. A summary of 42 studies concluded that participation in a walking group helped lower blood pressure, total cholesterol, body fat, and BMI.[45]

I recommend tracking your activity. You can go as simple or fancy as you like. A pedometer is an inexpensive way to count your daily steps. An hour of walking is about 10,000 steps. Or you might want to get a fitness band or fitness watch that syncs with your smartphone. They all work, as long as you use them. And tracking your steps helps you get into and stay in a routine.

One word of caution. If you increase your exercise a lot by working out longer or harder, you might need to eat a little more. If you create too big a gap between what you're eating and how many calories you're burning, your body puts on the brakes and preserves itself by holding on to every pound. If this happens to you, try moving to the Steady Loss meal plan.

What Are the Key Nutrients for Healthy Weight Loss?

While you may lose weight making swaps based purely on calorie counts, in the long term you may be depriving yourself of valuable nutrients and harming your health. You may also simply not find the lower-calorie options very satisfying. All of which means that way of eating is not sustainable, and you'll eventually revert to your old patterns.

Instead, in order to create lasting weight loss (and lasting good health), it's important to know which nutrients to stop eating and which to start eating. If you've read any of my previous books, you'll find these lists familiar.

▶ Ingredients to Stop Eating

In addition to calories, the top three numbers you should review on a nutrition label are these belly-bloating, health-harming ingredients:

- **Saturated and trans fats,** which can raise your cholesterol levels and fan the flames of inflammation. The 41,000-plus female participants in the Harvard University Nurses' Health Study were more likely to have gained weight over an 8-year period if their diet was higher in saturated and trans fats.[46]

- **Sodium,** which can raise your blood pressure and cause bloating. An Australian study found an association between eating more salty foods and drinking more sugar-sweetened beverages. Participants who consumed more than 1 serving of sugar-sweetened beverages were 26 percent more likely to be overweight or obese.[47]

- **Added sugars and other refined carbs,** which can raise your blood sugar and add extra calories. Although research findings have not been consistent, some experts suggest that extra calories from sugary drinks pack on the pounds.[48]

▶ Ingredients to Start Eating

The choices that Mindy and I recommend are high in health-protecting, tummy-trimming nutrients, including:

- **Lean protein** to keep your metabolism humming and your muscles strong. Plenty of evidence stresses the importance of eating enough protein when you're losing weight. At McMaster University in Hamilton, Ontario, Canada, dieters on a high-protein, high-dairy diet lost more fat and gained more muscle than those eating less protein and dairy.[49] Researchers in the Netherlands also found that dieters who ate the most protein while losing weight simultaneously increased their muscle mass.[50] Protein appears to aid weight loss and muscle health by stimulating hormones that make you feel full, boosting calorie burning, and helping keep blood sugar steady.[51]

- **Fiber** to keep your stomach full and your digestive tract in good health. Foods high in fiber, namely fruits, vegetables, whole grains, and legumes, are healthier and more filling than many other types of foods. A group of researchers at Columbia University compared a high-fiber oatmeal breakfast with low-fiber cornflakes to see which was more filling. Participants felt more full and less hungry after the oatmeal breakfast and also ate less at their next meal.[52]

- **Monounsaturated fatty acids** (MUFAs) to help you shed dangerous visceral belly fat. I've been raving about the tummy-slimming effects of MUFAs since I discovered them when writing my first book, *Flat Belly Diet!* A growing number of studies show that MUFAs, found in nuts, olive oil, avocadoes, and dark chocolate, appear to boost metabolism, increase the body's burning of calories and fat, and aid weight loss.[53] Also, people on a high-MUFA diet gained back less body fat and had lower risk factors for diabetes and heart disease.[54]

- **Calcium** to speed up your metabolism and burn more calories. In the multiyear Framingham Heart Study of more than 3,000 participants, people who included the most dairy in their diets gained less weight and fewer inches around their waist over a 17-year period.[55] Dairy products and fortified nondairy milks offer the most concentrated amounts of calcium in your diet, but you can also get calcium from leafy greens and nuts and seeds.

- **Vitamin C** to boost your immune system and your fat loss. People who are deficient in vitamin C may have a harder time shedding not only colds but also pounds. While it's not entirely clear why, the bodies of folks with inadequate levels of vitamin C seem to cling tight to fat.[56]

▶ Putting It All Together

In Part Three of this book, you'll find more than 700 foods that you can start eating to drop the weight. In picking foods to include, Mindy and I were very careful to consider not just the calorie count but the nutrition provided by the thousands of packaged and restaurant foods out there. Not every food listed, though, provides a good amount of fiber, protein, MUFAs, calcium, or vitamin C. And you'll see that some are a little high in saturated or trans fats, added sugars, and especially sodium.

In my perfect world, all foods in restaurants and packages would be low in fat, high in fiber, filled with vegetables and fruits, and made with whole grains. Sadly, that's far from reality, although I have to say that the food landscape has improved over the past couple of years. In fact, my local Panera Bread now sells bowls made with whole grains, veggies, and protein! Because I believe in eating real food in real places, I looked for the best possible swaps for unhealthy foods in particular restaurants and in brands of packaged foods. Even if they don't meet all of my guidelines, they still are a better alternative that allows you to drop calories and eat nutritious food.

And remember that it's your calorie and nutrient intake over time that really matters. If you eat one food that's high calorie and provides little to no nutrition (corn chips, anyone?), that's not such a big deal as long as the rest of your meals are generally nutritious. If you eat one food that's high in protein but low in fiber, that's fine as long as you balance it out with a food that provides the fiber.

That's where the Stop & Drop meals come in. In all three stages of the meal plan, Mindy's choices not only slash calories but also give you the best nutrient balance to boost your energy, keep you satisfied, and protect against aging and disease. In every phase, the plan aims to provide:

- Approximately 60 g of protein
- At least 25 g of fiber
- Less than 2400 mg of sodium
- At least 75 mg of vitamin C
- Approximately 1000 mg of calcium

Plus, in Chapter 4, you'll learn how to construct your own meals that meet these parameters.

Can I Keep Losing Weight This Fast?

It seems so simple at first. Simply drop (or burn) calories and lose weight. And in the beginning, this works. The low calorie level of the Kickstart meals helps jump-start weight loss, so we suggest that you start with this plan for your first week or two. This is the point at which you will most likely drop a pound a day or maybe even more.

And, in case you were wondering, yes, this is perfectly safe, as long as you eat in a way that is nutritionally balanced, as you will in the Kickstart phase. A group of weight loss experts note in a review article that more rapid weight loss is linked to better long-term results.[57]

But after a while, you might notice that you stop losing weight. You may even gain back a pound or two. And even if you follow each meal to the letter—or maybe cut back even more on your calories in the hopes of seeing better results—the scale won't budge. This disheartening plateau is the result of your body freaking out about your new, lower-calorie lifestyle. While the Kickstart meal plan is by no means a starvation diet, your body may think it is and react by holding on to every pound it can. And as you lose weight, your body requires fewer calories to move around because it takes more calories to move a heavy object than a lighter one. Less calorie burning means fewer pounds dropped.

To avoid that diet downer, we recommend that after a week or so, you switch to Steady Loss meals and snacks. These offer about 1600 calories per day and allow for more variety in your meals, both of which can be more satisfying. Although your rate of weight loss may slow down at this calorie level, you will still get to your weight loss goal over the course of weeks or months.

This is what happened to Diane Rohan, who, after dropping more than a pound a day in the first 5 days, suddenly found that she was gaining back weight in Week 2, even though she had actually cut back on her calories by skipping meals and cranking up her activity level. After she added in some Steady Loss meals, she started to lose again, shedding 3 more pounds by Day 12.

How Do I Keep the Weight Off for Good?

Once you've reached your weight loss goal, it's easy to slip back into your old eating habits. This is when it's critical that you remember to stop and think before putting anything into your mouth. "At my daughter's birthday party, I'm including turkey sandwiches, brownie-strawberry-marshmallow kebabs, and veggies!" Karen Woytach shared with us. "I can stay within my allotted calories by having only one snack that day." Because real life is full of temptations (the cheesy pasta at the office potluck, the chocolate cake at the birthday party) and challenges (the limited food choices when traveling, the rush to grab a fast meal in the morning), you must learn to make the best choices you can under any circumstances.

That's why we also offer a 2000-calorie-a-day Maintain meal plan. At this calorie level, you have a lot more choices, especially at restaurants and other settings where it can be tough to find healthy foods. Throughout the book, you may be surprised at some of the foods that are tagged for the Maintain phase, like IHOP Seasoned Fries (320 calories), Chick-fil-A Chick-n-Strips (360 calories), and a Dunkin' Donuts Jelly Donut (270 calories). With more calories to work with over the course of the day, you can have higher calorie, less nutritionally balanced food and still have enough calories to spare for healthful foods. This will help you keep the weight off for life.

Dropping pounds for good also requires you to stop behaviors that led to your weight gain in the first place and to continue weight-friendly behaviors that you started. As I mentioned earlier, one of the best guides to successful weight maintenance is the National Weight Control Registry, a database of several thousand people who lost at least 30 pounds and kept the weight off for at least one year. Among successful losers who maintained their loss for at least 10 years, the average weight loss was close to 70 pounds after 1 year, 53 after 5 years, and 51 after 10 years. Participants who gained back weight were less physically active, didn't stick to their diet, increased their calories from fat, and weighed themselves less often.[58]

In the British BeWEL study, participants who were most successful at losing weight over the course of a year ate more fruits and vegetables, did not let physical or emotional stumbling blocks get in the way of their routine, incorporated behavior changes into their lifestyle, and came up with strategies to help them deal with setbacks.[59] So maintaining your hard-earned loss calls for following an eating plan, walking or exercising nearly every day, and staying on top of your weight so that you can stop whatever behaviors are causing you to gain before you gain too much.

That's exactly what we recommend on the Stop & Drop Diet; it's how *you* will finally keep the weight off.

Chapter 3
WHAT MAKES THIS THE EASIEST DIET EVER

Now you've seen how the Stop & Drop Diet delivers fast—and lasting—weight loss results. But because no weight loss plan will work if you don't actually follow it, I was also determined to make sure that the plan is simple to understand and easy to use.

That's why I asked Mindy to create lists of quick, easy, and delicious breakfasts, lunches, dinners, and snacks to mix and match. You'll find these in Part Two. In putting together the meals, Mindy and I thought about all the different shopping and dining challenges we've encountered over the past 20 years of counseling dieters. We made sure the meals included everyday brand-name foods—no exotic, expensive, and hard-to-find herbs, berries, grains, or supplements. Then we included a variety of eat-in, eat-out, and grab-and-go meals so that you could follow the diet anywhere—even at airports, convenience stores, or fast-food restaurants. And we designed meals at different calorie levels that work equally well for people who have 10 pounds to lose or 100 pounds to lose, or even just for people who want to make healthier choices throughout the day.

Then we asked our testers to try them out. Guess what? They asked for more and told me how much they appreciated my planning out their meals for them. I took away the guesswork, and eating healthfully became easy and enjoyable. "I have definitely found a new way of eating!" exclaimed Karen Woytach. "I have my go-to and favorite meals and stick to what I know and like." Nora Healy enthused, "I spend a lot of time in the car and pass by Starbucks, Wendy's, McDonald's. Before this program, I would have looked at the signs and thought I CAN'T eat anything here. Now there are several places that I COULD eat, and that's a good feeling."

Once they got the hang of the meals, though, many of our testers wanted some variety. So in Part Three, we researched additional foods that you can use to customize your meals or make your own. Look for the foods or dishes you want to eat, from oatmeal to turkey sandwiches to spaghetti. You'll see at a glance the unhealthy versions you should stop eating and the lower-calorie, higher-nutrition options you should start eating instead. If a dish typically includes dressings, toppings, or condiments, we give you calorie counts for the most common options so that you can personalize it. Now let's take a closer look at how incredibly easy, flexible, and convenient the Stop & Drop Diet is.

It Uses Everyday Foods and Brands

One of my earliest memories as a little girl was coming home from Sunview School at lunchtime. Mom and I would sit at the kitchen table by the window, and I'd tell her about the books we'd read in class and which friends had been nice to me that day while she cracked open a box of Kraft Macaroni & Cheese for us to share. While I've since enjoyed gourmet pastas, to this day, I still occasionally crave a little Kraft Mac & Cheese.

Luckily, on the Stop & Drop Diet, I can have some. I can also have my favorite cereal (Kix), grab my usual salad (a half-size Panera Fuji Apple Chicken Salad), and even enjoy an occasional dessert (a half cup of Breyers Triple Chocolate Gelato Indulgences). In choosing the foods and dishes to include, Mindy made sure to consider restaurants and brands that are available nationwide or at least in broad regions. She looked for dishes that were low enough in calories (often on the kids' or lunch menus) to allow for other foods to round out the meal. For example, she spotted the 240-calorie Panda Express Shanghai Angus Steak from the kids' menu and paired it with a side order of mixed veggies and a partial portion of brown rice to create a 413-calorie Steady Loss meal.

That being said, of course, your local grocery store may not have all the items on the list in stock. And, while we did our very best to fact-check and update all the foods featured in the book, food manufacturers frequently discontinue items and restaurants change their menus. If that's the case, don't panic! You'll find more guidance on how to make substitutions as necessary in Chapter 4.

You Can Do It Anywhere, Anytime

It's easy to be good on a diet when you have the time to plan out all your meals and your shopping lists, cook enough to make hearty, healthy leftovers, and research any restaurants you might visit ahead of time. But life is rarely that obliging. The kids beg for pizza, your boss drags you out to a steakhouse for a last-minute business dinner, and your spouse insists on hitting every drive-through on your family's summer road trip. The true test of any diet is whether you can follow it anywhere life takes you.

The Stop & Drop Diet is designed so you can do just that. Family wants pizza? Turn to the pizza page in Chapter 12, Main Dishes, and offer to bake Newman's Own Thin & Crispy Uncured Pepperoni Pizza and eat just a third of it (the kids will polish off the rest!). Or order a medium 12-inch Pizza Hut Veggie Lover's pan pizza so you can get the kids to eat their veggies, too. At a steakhouse with clients? Check out the steak page in Chapter 12. Go for a 6-ounce sirloin and skip the calorie-laden sides that come with the steak. Ask for mixed steamed vegetables instead. At the Burger King drive-through? Flip through Chapter 11, Sandwiches, and you'll see you can opt for the TENDERGRILL Chicken Sandwich (order it without mayo) or the Whopper Jr. (you can have mayo on this one, if you'd like, or leave it off for even more calorie savings—100 calories for every tablespoon).

Our testers agreed that the Stop & Drop Diet helped them navigate some of these common diet challenges. "I was running around like a mad-woman and at 2:30 hadn't had a chance to eat lunch yet. I had to grab something quick and decided to get the cheeseburger meal from Wendy's. As I was eating it, I kept thinking to myself . . . YOU'RE CHEATING!!! But I wasn't!" celebrated Karen Woytach. Donna Lindskog reported, "On a recent business trip, my boss was dying for fried chicken. So we went to a restaurant with fried chicken but I ordered grilled instead."

And if you do have time to plan and cook more, all the better. You'll also find quick, five-ingredient recipes to lighten up your favorite lunches and dinners, plus the best choices for frozen and packaged foods to keep on hand to help build your Stop & Drop meals.

It Works No Matter How Much You Have to Lose

Do you have 50 or more pounds to lose? The Stop & Drop Diet is made for you. The Kickstart phase will reeducate your brain, your eyes, and your stomach about proper portions while its lower calorie level will help you shed pounds quickly. Again, how much you lose depends on a lot of factors, but the heavier you are, the more likely you are to drop a lot at first because people who have higher amounts of body fat lose body fat more rapidly when they cut calories.

What if, like me, you only have 10 pounds or so to lose? The last 5 pounds are the hardest to lose because, as your body gets smaller, the number of calories it burns drops. And I already ate relatively healthfully and exercised regularly. So I was skeptical that the small changes I was making in the Stop & Drop Diet could make a difference. But I dropped 2 pounds in just the first day of the Kickstart! Sure, my weight loss slowed after that, but I still took 8¼ inches off my waist in the 3 weeks of the diet.

Remember, small changes do add up over time. And while you may have been sticking to a reasonable calorie intake on a regular basis, it's possible that some tummy-troubling ingredients like added sugars have snuck by you. People typically say that they've eaten less than they actually have, and it's hard to keep track of every gram of sugar or fat.[60] Or you may have unknowingly been shorting yourself of nutrients like calcium and fiber that can help you lose weight. Our average fiber intake, for example, falls about 10 grams short of the amount that's recommended.[61]

What if weight isn't really your problem (lucky you!)? The Stop & Drop Diet can still help you to make healthier choices at the supermarket, at the fast-food counter, and in the restaurant. That will help you keep the weight off and feel better.

You Can Tailor the Meals to Work for You

When we first showed our list of meals to our testers, a number of people said to us, "But I never go to fast-food restaurants! Having a Wendy's cheeseburger seems like it would be going backward!" Once upon a time, I would have thought so, too, but as I mentioned in Chapter 1, I was pleasantly surprised to find that many fast-food restaurants now offer more lower-calorie, lower-fat options. That being said, if you really don't want to have a Wendy's cheeseburger, don't have one! Or if you fear that as soon as you walk into Wendy's, you'll feel compelled to order the fries along with the burger, skip it. We offer the Wendy's cheeseburger on the Kickstart meal plan for people who want it or for people who may find themselves in a place where fast food is the only option (at a rest stop or an airport, for instance). But remember that you are NOT required to eat all or any of the specific meals. Just choose the meals that appeal to you.

Same goes for any packaged foods. You may be surprised to see some chips and cookies and sodas among the foods featured in Part Three. We've included them so that you can enjoy your favorite treats once in a while because I firmly believe that no foods should be forbidden. I don't know about you, but if I'm told I can never have a brownie again, having a brownie is all I think about. It's just human nature. But if you're worried that once you start eating these foods, you won't be able to stop at the portion indicated, then skip them!

And what if there's a food you just don't like in a given meal? There's no need to eat it. Simply choose a different meal from the list. Or, check out Chapter 4 to see how you can make substitutions for certain meal components. Say, for instance, you really like the sound of Kickstart Dinner #7 (baked tilapia with clam chowder and steamed broccoli) but you can't stand broccoli. Check out the "Vegetable Swaps" chart on page 59 to see what other veggies you can have instead—zucchini, green beans, peppers, or mushrooms. You can also swap vegetables if you happen to have extra green beans you want to use up.

You Can Feed Your Family, Too

If you're single, you call the shots on what to eat. But throw a spouse and/or kids into the mix, and suddenly you have a whole other diet challenge. It's really hard to stick to a diet if you have one lonely little grilled skinless chicken breast on your plate while the rest of your family is tucking into a big bucket of KFC extra-crispy chicken with mashed potatoes and gravy.

That's why I asked Mindy to ensure that, first, all the meals are filling and delicious. You'll never have just a plain grilled chicken breast for dinner, I promise! However, you might fall in love with the simple chicken breast sautéed with 1 cup sliced mushrooms and served with Uncle Ben's Ready Rice Whole Grain Brown Rice and Progresso Vegetable Classics Vegetarian Vegetable with Barley Soup (that's Kickstart Dinner #2).

Second, all the meals are family friendly, so you don't have to cook one thing for yourself and something else for your family. And, in doing so, you'll have the satisfaction of knowing that you've provided everyone with a healthy and nutritious meal. "I made a taco lasagna for my family and used the same ingredients to make my Stop & Drop meal," said Nora Healy. "I felt like I was eating the same thing my family was eating." Tester Carol Maymudes revealed, "My shopping changed because I learned that I was buying the wrong foods. Now I'm making things I never used to eat, like sautéed spinach with garlic, and my husband is losing weight, too!"

You Decide How Much to Change

Finally, no diet will work unless and until you're truly committed to making a change. For some of you, the Stop & Drop meals may feel like a radical departure from the way you're eating now. For others, it's just a matter of small tweaks. With the Stop & Drop Diet, you can decide how much you're comfortable changing and when. If you're used to eating out at every meal and supersizing them all, you may decide to stick with the restaurant meals in the Maintain meal plan. Or, if you want to make a bigger change, you could jump in with the Kickstart meals and pick as many of the home-cooked meals as possible. Either way, you'll be making a change that will benefit your waist, your heart, and your whole body. Now let's get started!

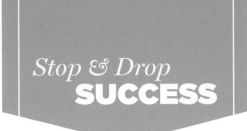
Angela Mastrantuono, a construction accountant, knew that she needed to get healthier by eating better and losing weight. She had successfully lost 50 pounds three years earlier and was thrilled that her various health problems disappeared. She felt great! Then life's challenges, including a new job and illness in the family, got in the way and Angela's healthy habits went by the wayside. She fell back into eating a lot of carbs, snacking without focusing on what she was eating, and not exercising. All of her lost pounds eventually came back.

"This plan is the wake-up call I needed!"

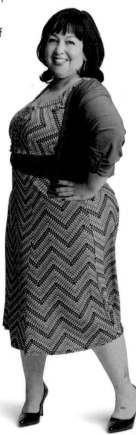

"I kept telling myself that I would start tomorrow, but one day I realized I couldn't do that anymore. I needed to fall in love again with working out, being healthy, loving my body, and taking care of myself. I felt depressed, lacking, and in need of rehab. I've known and trusted Reader's Digest for my whole life and want to be on a plan that doesn't have to end. Heathy habits need to be in my head."

Angela lost 8 pounds in the first 5 days. But even more meaningful is the change in the way she feels. "My mood and energy have increased. I am much more conscious of what I put in my mouth. I thought tracking my food would annoy me, but it woke me up to the fact that I was always eating but never was satisfied. This plan is the wake-up call that I needed.

"The plan also got me back to food shopping, and that relieved tension because I always knew what I would be eating for the next day. Another benefit that I am gaining . . . but in the right place—my wallet! It is so nice to bring lunch from home and not have to instead spend a lot of money to wind up with something that is bad for me. I feel enlightened, restarted, and determined. I am eating what I should be eating."

Part Two
THE **DIET** AND **MEAL PLANS**

You'll find everything you need to know to follow the Stop & Drop Diet here in Part Two. First I'll explain how the three phases work, answer common questions about the diet, and describe how you can customize the meals to suit your tastes. Then, you'll see all the Stop & Drop meals that you can choose from. Within each phase, the meals are listed roughly by type—that is, egg-based breakfasts are grouped together, as are lunch salads, pasta dinners, salty snacks, and so on. We've illustrated one of each type of meal to show the exact proportions of the meal components. This will help you train your eye, as well as your stomach, to recognize what a nutritionally balanced and calorically correct Stop & Drop meal looks like.

Chapter 4
MAKE THE STOP & DROP MEALS WORK FOR YOU

Good news! It's time to start talking about my favorite subject: food. In this chapter, I'll detail exactly what you need to do on the Stop & Drop Diet for maximum results in the minimum amount of time.

The Stop & Drop Phases— And How to Adapt Them

First, a word about words. The word *diet*, as I frequently note, does not just mean "a short period of calorie restriction designed to cause weight loss," even though that's what many of us have come to associate it with. The word can also refer to what you eat on a regular basis—your way of eating, in other words. To that point, I hope you'll find the Stop & Drop Diet a way of eating that you can stick to for life.

In fact, that's what we recommend. The Stop & Drop Diet has three phases: Kickstart, Steady Loss, and Maintain. On each phase, you'll find a menu of meals to choose from that includes a mix of packaged foods, restaurant meals, and quick and easy recipes so that you can stop eating mindlessly and start making smart choices to drop the pounds.

The difference between the three phases? Calories. For most of you, here's what your Stop & Drop Diet will look like:

Phase	Calories per day	Duration
Kickstart	1200	1 week
Steady Loss	1600	2 weeks or until you reach your goal weight*
Maintain	2000	The rest of your life

*Alternatively, you can cycle between 1 week of Kickstart and 2 weeks of Steady Loss until you reach your goal weight.

The chart outlines the plan our testers followed—or, I suppose I should say, are still following! Because we had to stop conducting weigh-ins in order to get the book done, we only assessed everybody for 3 weeks. But they tell me they're still maintaining and enjoying their Stop & Drop meals!

The structured Stop & Drop phases happen to be the best way to lose the most weight in the least amount of time. Kickstart takes pounds off quickly at first. The Steady Loss phase introduces more calories to help you avoid plateaus and more meals to keep you interested so you don't drop off from boredom or cravings. You will still lose weight, even if not as quickly. How long you stay on Steady Loss depends, of course, on how much weight you want to lose. It might be just a month or two; it might be a year.

During this time, if you need more variety, you can cycle back through Kickstart every 2 weeks. Or you can mix and match meals from the different phases. If you find a Kickstart snack you love, feel free to have it during your Steady Loss phase. If a Steady Loss breakfast is especially convenient, by all means have it during a Kickstart week. You can even enjoy an occasional Maintain meal if you have a craving for chicken fingers or cake.

Once you've reached your goal weight, move on to the Maintain phase. As its name implies, this phase was designed to help you maintain your hard-won weight loss. At 2000 calories, this level allows for some "treat" foods that are not as nutritious so that you never feel deprived. That makes it easy to enjoy this phase for life.

For some folks, though, a different timetable may be optimal. If you:

- **Want to lose weight for a specific event coming up,** stay on Kickstart for up to 3 weeks before you switch to Steady Loss.

- **Get at least 30 minutes of moderately intense exercise (like walking briskly or bicycling leisurely) or 20 minutes of vigorous activity (like running or Spinning) on most days of the week,** try Kickstart for just 3 days. Then switch to Steady Loss.

- **Are taller than 6 feet,** try Kickstart for just 3 days. Then switch to Steady Loss.

- **Are obese,** look over the three plans and find the one that is closest to the way you eat now in terms of amount of food. If you eat more than the Maintain plan, start on that plan. If Maintain is closer to your current diet, then start on Steady Loss. You should work with your doctor, dietitian, and/or personal trainer to fine-tune your diet as you lose weight.

- **Lose more than 2 pounds a day on Kickstart** or feel faint or nauseous, totally zapped of energy, and/or unable to concentrate on Kickstart, stop and switch to Steady Loss.

How Do I Know What My Goal Weight Should Be?

Most of us have a goal weight in mind, but do you know if yours is realistic? You might dream about being the same weight as you were in high school, but if you were a scrawny kid and now you're strong and fit, that number might be too low to be healthy. Most of us should aim to stay within the normal body mass index (BMI) range, a widely used measure of body fat. Look it up at www.cdc.gov/healthyweight/assessing/bmi/adult_bmi/english_bmi_calculator/bmi_calculator.html.

Six Stop & Drop Diet Fundamentals

These guidelines apply to all three phases of the Stop & Drop Diet:

1) Choose from the lists of breakfasts, lunches, dinners, and snacks provided. Lunches and dinners within each of the three phases have similar calories, so feel free to have a lunch at dinner and vice versa. On Kickstart, you'll have one snack per day; on Steady Loss and Maintain, you can have two.

2) Eat meals approximately 4 hours apart and don't go more than 5 hours without eating. You can split any meal into two minimeals, if you prefer to eat more frequently.

3) Follow the meals as closely as possible. If you do not consume dairy products, substitute calcium-fortified, unsweetened almond milk, light soy milk, or calcium-fortified juice for dairy milk, and non-dairy cheeses for cheese. If you are vegetarian, simply stick to the vegetarian options in the lists.

4) Walk an hour or more a day. These can be four 15-minute walks or shorter if needed. If you already have a regular exercise routine, keep it up and add walking on top of that. The results will astound you.

5) Keep track of your eating, activity, and hunger levels on paper, on the computer, or with a phone app. People who write down what they eat find it easier to stick with an eating plan.

6) While you're on the Kickstart and Steady Loss phases, Mindy recommends taking a multivitamin that provides 100% of the Daily Value for most vitamins and minerals. If you are a postmenopausal woman, choose an iron-free formulation. Additionally, most women should take a daily calcium supplement of at least 600 mg while on this eating plan. Reputable supplement brands include Nature Made, Centrum, Kirkland, Trader Joe's, 365 Everyday Value, and Whole Foods Market. You can also get your calcium from a calcium carbonate antacid such as Tums.

Swap & Drop FAQs

I designed the Stop & Drop Diet to be flexible, but there are some guidelines that will help you lose weight safely and quickly. Where there are rules, there are questions! Here are the most common ones that came up when I tested the diet with our panelists.

▶ Meals

Q: Should I eat at set mealtimes?

A: Set mealtimes are not necessary, but it's best to eat meals approximately 4 hours apart. And try to allow no more than 5 hours between meals.

....

Q: Can I eat the same meals each day?

A: From a calorie standpoint, you can eat the same meals each day. However, optimal nutrition comes from variety, so I encourage you to try as many different meals as possible.

....

Q: Do I have to buy the specific brands and products listed in the meal plans and recipes?

A: Please try to, yes. Mindy and I have selected particular brands because of their taste, quality, availability, and nutritional value, including calorie level. In Part Three, you'll notice that we recommend certain brands and products to stop eating and others to start. I asked Mindy to research thousands of foods, brands, and restaurant meals to tease out subtle differences that make some lower in calories and higher in nutrients than others.

....

Q: Can I pick any combination of meals I like?

A: Yes. But while the plan is designed so that you don't need to count calories, it's best to be aware of your overall calorie intake. So if you pick one of the higher-calorie breakfasts in each phase, go for one of the lower-calorie lunches or dinners to keep your daily calories at around the correct level.

....

Q: Do I need to make the meals exactly as shown?

A: As long as you are eating all the components of a meal, it doesn't matter how you put them together. For instance, in Steady Loss Breakfast #3, we've created a parfait with ¾ cup Kashi GOLEAN Crunch!, 1 carton Dannon Oikos Plain Nonfat Greek Yogurt, and 1 small cubed pear. But if you don't like the way these flavors work together, or you're in too much of a hurry to cut up the pear, or you want to eat part of the meal before your morning walk and part of it after, you can choose instead to eat the cereal, the yogurt, and the pear all separately. Or mix the cereal with the yogurt and eat the pear later. Or whatever other combination you choose.

Q: Can I pair the side dishes from one meal with the entrée from another? That way I'll have more varied lunch and dinner options.

A: You can swap side dishes as long as they are similar—for example, broccoli instead of green beans or pasta instead of rice. Check out the charts on pages 56–59 for more ideas on changing one food for another.

Q: Can I serve Kickstart meals to my family? I don't want to make two sets of meals.

A: Kickstart foods are perfectly healthy and appealing for families, but you might want to increase portions, depending on your family members' calorie needs.

Q: I usually have a shake or smoothie for breakfast. Can I keep doing that?

A: Many ready-made shakes and smoothies are surprisingly high in calories. Try one of the Kickstart smoothie recipes instead!

Q: Some of the meals call for an olive oil spray. I've never used one before. Which do you recommend?

A: I like Pam or Bertolli olive oil spray. Or you can put olive oil into a sprayer/mister such as Misto.

▶ Foods

Q: Is it important for me to measure my food?

A: For best results, I suggest that you measure or weigh the food in your plan as frequently as possible, and as a rule for the first week or two. It's very easy to accumulate extra calories by eyeballing portions, especially when we "forget" the right sizes as time goes by. When you're not at home, it can be difficult to measure everything. At those times, having read the "Portion Guide" on page 9 will come in handy.

Q: Can I add salt or other seasonings?

A: You can add a few shakes of salt to food, but please limit your intake. While salt has no calories, it does contribute to bloat, which can add inches and pounds. Instead, use herbs, spices, and other seasonings with fewer than 5 calories per serving.

Q: Can I make substitutions?

A: Refer to the charts on pages 56–59 for ways to swap fixings for cereals, sandwiches, and salads, and also proteins, side dishes, fruits, and vegetables. In beverages, you may substitute almond or soy products for dairy products, as long as they provide a similar number of calories and are fortified with calcium.

....

Q: I see a lot of red "Stop" signs in Part Three. Do you really mean that I should stop eating certain foods? I thought you said no foods were forbidden!

A: The foods labeled "Stop Eating" in Part Three are higher in calories (and/or in fattening ingredients like saturated fat and sugars) than their counterparts that we say to "Start Eating." Switch away from the higher-calorie option so you trim calories without making major changes in what you eat.

....

Q: I see a lot of branded choices. I don't eat much fast food or packaged foods. Are you telling me I have to start eating them now?

A: I've included fast food and packaged foods in the meal plans in Part Two (as well as in Part Three) because I know how many people need (or want) the convenience they provide. But you don't have to eat them. There are plenty of cook-at-home options for you to choose from instead.

....

Q: Are all of the "Start Eating" foods good for me?

A: Not necessarily. Throughout Part Three, you'll find foods that you might not expect to see in a weight loss book. I included them because I wanted to help people deal with the real food situations that come up in their lives. A Super Bowl party, for example, will likely have chips and chili. Halloween means candy at home and in the office. The Stop & Drop Diet educates you so you know how to make good choices wherever you are, whatever your real-life eating challenges.

....

Q: Can I eat candies, drinks, or other products with artificial sweeteners?

A: I don't like artificial sweeteners, and science has conflicting things to say about their health effects. In general, it's best just to eat fewer sweets. But on those occasions when you really have a craving for a soda, mint, or gum, then a zero-calorie option may be best. You'll find a few of them in Part Three.

....

▶ Drinks

Q: What can I drink on the Stop & Drop Diet?

A: Any noncaloric beverages are fine, including water (flavored with a lemon slice or other fresh fruit, if desired), sparkling water, coffee, and tea. When drinking coffee and tea, just be careful not to overdo it with milk or other add-ins—you might want to "borrow" milk from another meal or snack to use in your drink. And, as I just noted, while I'm not a fan myself, you may have diet sodas, teas, or other drinks made with noncaloric sweeteners. You'll see that there are other drinks listed in Chapter 16, Drinks. These are fine to have occasionally, but most drinks give you very little nutrition for a lot of calories, so it's best not to have them at every meal.

....

Q: What about cappuccinos, lattes, and other coffee or tea drinks?

A: You can substitute a small-size coffee or tea drink made with fat-free milk in place of a serving of milk or yogurt on the menu. Drinks should preferably be unsweetened, but you may use a noncaloric sweetener or syrup.

Q: Is a beer or glass of wine OK?

A: Yes, you can enjoy a 12-oz glass of beer or 6-oz glass of wine in place of a snack once or twice a week. Remember, though, while beer and wine may be equivalent to your snack calorie-wise, the snacks add nutrients and will keep you fuller longer, so you don't want to make this swap every day.

▶ Activity

Q: Do I have to exercise?

A: For the best weight loss results, yes, you should walk 1 hour or more each day. You can break this up into several smaller walks to fit it in. Exercise not only burns calories but also builds muscle tissue, which has a faster metabolism than fat tissue does.

Q: What if I am completely sedentary now but have gotten my doctor's okay to do this plan?

A: Work up to walking 1 hour a day. On Day 1, start with just one 15-minute walk at a pace that feels modestly challenging to you. The next day, add a second 15-minute walk. By Day 4, you'll be walking 1 hour a day! After you've gotten used to walking, you can gradually increase your pace so that you're burning more calories in less time.

Q: I have a fitness tracker. What's the 1-hour equivalent in terms of steps?

A: It depends on how quickly you walk, but if you are walking briskly, in 1 hour most people will walk about 10,000 steps—which, for people with average strides, is about 5 miles.

Q: What's the best way to time meals and exercise?

A: Try to eat a snack 60 to 90 minutes before you exercise. You may want to eat your next meal soon after, if you are hungry.

Q: I find walking boring. Can I do something else?

A: Absolutely! I jump on a trampoline with my kids, do yoga, and take the occasional Zumba class. I recommend walking because almost everyone can do it, you can do it anywhere, and it requires no special equipment. But any movement burns calories, gets your heart rate up, builds your lean muscle mass, and protects against disease. Try fitness classes, strength training, dancing, biking, swimming, vigorous gardening, or whatever else you enjoy. The key is to move and to do so every day.

Q: I didn't have time to walk today, but I shoveled snow/cleaned the house/played with my kids. Does that count, or do I still need to walk an hour on top of that?

A: All movement counts! But not all activity burns an equal number of calories as walking. See the chart on page 53 to get an idea of how different kinds of activity stack up, and mix and match as you like. Remember, the more you move, the more calories you burn, and the faster you'll lose weight.

▶ Shopping and Dining

Q: I can't find a particular item for a meal in the grocery store. What do I do?

A: Don't panic! Check out the corresponding food page in Part Three and select the alternative that's closest in calorie count. Or look for a similar item that has 20 calories more or less than the item in the meal plan.

For example, many of our testers (me included!) had trouble finding the Good Food Made Simple Chicken Apple Sausage Egg White Breakfast Burrito (310 calories) on the Kickstart meal plan. If you can't find it either, check out the Breakfast Sandwiches and Wraps page in Chapter 8, Breakfast Foods (yes, after my husband's misadventures on his first shopping trip, I brought the book with me to the store for the first couple of weeks!). You'll see that you can try any of these alternatives:

- Jimmy Dean Delights Bacon, Egg & Cheese Honey Wheat Flatbread (230 calories)
- Amy's Breakfast Burrito (270 calories)
- Weight Watchers Smart Ones Smart Beginnings Canadian Style Turkey Bacon English Muffin Sandwich (210 calories)
- Atkins Canadian Bacon with Egg and Cheese English Muffin Sandwich (230 calories)
- Amy's Southwestern Burrito (290 calories)
- Good Food Made Simple Turkey Sausage Breakfast Burrito (300 calories)

You want to find the alternative that's closest in calorie count to the original choice—in this case, that means you want to look first for the Good Food Made Simple Turkey Sausage Breakfast Burrito. If you don't have your book with you at the store, try to find another breakfast sandwich or wrap that's between 290 and 330 calories.

Q: What if a restaurant is no longer serving the dish that's listed on the meal plan?

A: Choose another of our meal options from the same restaurant, if possible. If there is no other meal option from that restaurant, then try to construct a meal for yourself that mimics the MyPlate recommendations I mentioned in Chapter 1—that is, something that's approximately one-quarter protein, one-quarter grain, and half vegetable and fruit. Because restaurants often go heavy on the protein, you are likely to have leftover meat, which you can use to create another meal at home later.

And remember to choose the simplest dishes—that is, no sauces, gravies, or dressings. You never know how much fat or sugar the chef will put in them; chefs tend to have a heavy hand with butter, and they can add a couple hundred calories to your dish in just two or three tablespoons!

Q: What if I am eating all the meals and snacks, but I'm still hungry?

A: It is not unusual to feel hungry, especially during the first few days of the Kickstart. Try to drink noncaloric beverages when hunger hits. You can also divide up your meals so you're eating more frequently during the day. Tester Angela Mastrantuono found herself missing her late-night dessert, so instead of eating the sweet potato with Kickstart Dinner #11 (lean roast beef, sweet potato, greens, and cantaloupe), she saved it for dessert. That hit her sweet spot. If you are still really hungry, you can munch on raw or lightly steamed or boiled green vegetables. You might also try chewing sugar-free gum. While some studies have found its effects inconsistent,[62] others have found that chewing gum helps curb your appetite.[63]

Q: I have to eat out for business frequently. Can I still be on this plan?

A: Yes. This plan includes a lot of different options for eating out. If you are not eating at one of the chain restaurants mentioned in the book, you can look for or ask the restaurant to prepare a meal from the meal plan. (Many restaurants, for instance, would be able to prepare Kickstart Dinner #8 for you, which is 4 oz grilled salmon, 2 cups sautéed greens, and a small whole wheat roll.) Or follow the MyPlate recommendations in Chapter 1.

Q: What if I need to travel during the time I'm on this plan?

A: You can stay on the Stop & Drop Diet with a bit of advance preparation. Look through the meals to identify those that would be easy to find on the road. Several of our testers, including Donna Lindskog and Nora Healy, took the diet on the road, and were thrilled to report that they had no problems finding things to eat.

▶ Weight Loss and Nutrition

Q: My weight loss has really slowed. Am I doing something wrong?

A: No. Especially if you're heading into Weeks 2 or 3 of the plan, it's natural for weight loss to slow. Don't panic. Just start experimenting with varying your calorie levels a bit. If you've been on Kickstart for more than a week or two, try switching to or at least adding in some Steady Loss meals. If you've been on Steady Loss for more than a few days, it could be that 1600 calories is too high for you. Try incorporating one or two Kickstart meals into each day to lower the calories. Also be sure to walk at least 1 hour a day (more if you can), because exercise helps you burn calories and burst through plateaus.

Q: I've reached my goal weight. Now what?

A: Switch to the Maintain phase. If you start to gain weight within, say, 2 or 3 weeks, switch back to Steady Loss. Now that you weigh less, your body needs fewer calories, so 1600 might be just right for maintaining your weight. (If you happen to have reached your goal weight while on the Kickstart phase, switch to Steady Loss meals to maintain it.)

How Many Calories Can I Burn in 30 Minutes?

How many calories you burn doing different activities depends on a lot of different factors, but this table, adapted from one created by Harvard Health Publications, will give you an idea of approximate calories burned in 30 minutes for people of three different weights.[64] In each category, calories are listed from least to most calories burned.

Activities	125-pound person	155-pound person	185-pound person
Gym			
Weight lifting (general)	90	112	133
Stretching, hatha yoga	120	149	178
Aerobics (low impact)	165	205	244
Bicycling, stationary (moderate)	210	260	311
Elliptical trainer (general)	285	353	422
Training and Sport Activities			
Dancing (slow, waltz, fox-trot)	90	112	133
Golf (using cart)	105	130	155
Walking (3.5 mph)	120	149	178
Softball (general play)	150	186	222
Dancing (disco, ballroom, square)	180	223	266
Swimming (general)	180	223	266
Tennis (general)	210	260	311
Basketball (playing a game)	240	298	355
Running (5 mph)	240	298	355
Home and Daily Life Activities			
Food shopping (with cart)	105	130	155
Playing with kids (moderate effort)	120	149	178
Gardening (general)	135	167	200
Heavy cleaning (wash car, windows)	135	167	200
Shoveling snow (by hand)	180	223	266

Q: I am worried about the sodium levels in some of the meals, especially those with packaged foods. What should I do?

A: Sodium can be higher in convenience foods, but many packaged foods are much lower in sodium than they used to be. You might find lower sodium choices in the healthy food or organic section of the market. (But again, pay attention to the nutrition labels. Just because a product is labeled "lower sodium" doesn't mean it has the least sodium.) It's true that in some cases, we recommended a higher-sodium product (because it had fewer calories, saturated fat, and/or sugars). But for the most part, we still tried to keep sodium levels in check. Unless your doctor has recommended that you follow a low-salt diet, don't worry too much about sodium! If your doctor has recommended that you follow a low-salt diet, please share this diet with him or her first.

Q: Why do I need to take a multivitamin?

A: It is virtually impossible to meet the dietary recommendations for all vitamins and minerals on a higher-calorie diet, let alone one that is calorie restricted. While Mindy and I designed this eating plan to be nutritionally balanced, she recommends a multivitamin on the Kickstart and Steady Loss phases to help cover all nutrition bases.

Make Your Own Stop & Drop Meals

While we've given you a lot of meals to choose from, we know that you don't want to be restricted to eating from this list for the rest of your life. To that end, Mindy created swap charts for many of the components of the meals.

You can use these to customize the meals from the three meal plans. For instance, say you like the idea of Kickstart Dinner #12 (which includes sirloin steak, a baked potato, and green beans) but prefer rice and don't have green beans on hand. So, following the swap charts below, you can swap rice pilaf for your potato and broccoli for the green beans.

Alternatively, you can use these to create your own meals. I've included some charts to help you construct healthy cereal bowls, sandwiches, and salads. Or choose a protein, a side dish, and a vegetable from the charts below to make up your lunch or dinner plate. As you mix and match, keep these guidelines in mind:

For each day, you're aiming for:

- 1200 calories for Kickstart, 1600 calories for Steady Loss, and 2000 calories for Maintain

- Approximately 60 g of protein (include some at every meal and snack)

- At least 25 g of fiber

- Less than 2400 mg of sodium

- At least 75 mg of vitamin C

- Approximately 1000 mg of calcium from a combination of foods (each dairy serving provides about 300 mg) and a supplement

The calories and nutrients can be spread throughout the day in a number of different ways, but to get to the right numbers, here are some general guidelines Mindy used to construct the meals:

	Kickstart Meal Plan	Steady Loss Meal Plan	Maintain Meal Plan	Include These Types of Food
Breakfast	300 calories	350 calories	450 calories	Grain, fruit, dairy, and/or protein
Lunch & Dinner	350–400 calories	400–450 calories	525 calories	Vegetables, protein, grain, fruit, and/or dairy
Snack	1 x 150 calories	2 x 200 calories	2 x 250 calories	Fruit, vegetables, grain, and/or protein

You'll see, of course, that not all the meals in our plan fit these exact guidelines or even stay exactly within these calorie ranges (especially the snacks) because in the real world, not all foods fit into these neat categories. But this will provide you an easy formula to start with when creating your own meals. Don't go crazy counting calories and protein grams, for example, but use our guidelines to help you choose foods and ingredients.

▶ Basic Dish Generators

First, here are a few charts to help you create some basic dishes: a balanced cereal bowl for breakfast, and healthy sandwiches and salads for lunches and dinners. These were staples for our testers, so we wanted to make it especially easy to mix and match for simple, hearty meals.

Note that the foods in these charts do range quite a bit in calories, so be sure to pay attention to portions and read labels to figure out how many calories your favorite combinations contain. In some cases, you'll need to add some additional foods to these dishes to round out your meals. If you mix together ½ cup Kellogg's All-Bran Original (80 calories) with 1 cup fat-free milk (83 calories) and ½ cup strawberries (27 calories), for instance, you will have a 190-calorie cereal bowl. If you're on Kickstart, that means you can have another 110 calories or so worth of food, so you might want to add yogurt or some nuts for more protein. On Steady Loss, you could add about 160 calories, perhaps with an egg or a small piece of cheese and some fruit. On Maintain, when you could have another 260 calories, you might be able to add all of these.

Cereal Bowl Generator

Pick one from each column.

Cereal	Dairy / Nondairy	Fruit
¾ cup Kellogg's All-Bran Complete Wheat Flakes (90 calories)	1 cup calcium-fortified almond or soy milk (up to 80 calories)	½ cup strawberries (27 calories)
1¼ cups Kix (110 calories)	1 5.2–6 oz 0% plain Greek or light fat-free yogurt (80–100 calories)	½ cup sliced peaches (30 calories)
1 cup Cascadian Farm Honey Nut O's (110 calories)	1 cup fat-free milk (83 calories)	½ cup raspberries (32 calories)
¾ cup Kellogg's All-Bran Original (120 calories)		½ cup fresh blueberries (42 calories)
¾ cup Life (120 calories)		½ small banana (45 calories)
¾ cup Wheat Chex (160 calories)		

Sandwich Generator

Pick one from each column below, then add up to ½ cup raw veggies of your choice (lettuce, tomato, onion, bell pepper, roasted red pepper, shredded carrots, etc.) for only 20 extra calories.

Bread	Protein	Spread
Pepperidge Farm Very Thin 100% Whole Wheat (2 slices) (72 calories)	3 oz turkey breast (78 calories)	1 tsp honey mustard (12 calories)
Thomas' Light Multi-Grain English Muffin (100 calories)	4 oz shaved roast beef (133 calories)	1 Tbsp mustard (15 calories)
Flatout 100% Whole Wheat (100 calories)	3 oz grilled chicken breast (140 calories)	2 tsp hummus (20 calories)
Thomas' 100% Whole Wheat Bagel Thin (110 calories)	1½ Tbsp peanut butter (141 calories)	2 tsp reduced-fat mayonnaise (22 calories)
Arnold Stone Ground 100% Whole Wheat Bread (2 slices) (130 calories)	4 oz deli ham (148 calories)	1 Tbsp light Italian dressing (40 calories)
	2 1-oz slices reduced-fat cheese (160 calories)	2 tsp guacamole (57 calories)

Salad Generator

Pick one from each column below, then add up to 1 cup raw veggies of your choice (tomato, onion, carrot, bell pepper, broccoli, cauliflower, etc.) for up to 40 extra calories.

Greens (2 cups)	Protein	Dressing
Arugula (10 calories)	3 oz water-packed tuna (73 calories)	1 Tbsp 0% plain Greek yogurt (8 calories)
Spinach (14 calories)	3 oz turkey breast (78 calories)	1 Tbsp light Miracle Whip (20 calories)
Lettuce (15 calories)	3 oz grilled chicken breast (140 calories)	1 Tbsp reduced-fat ranch (30 calories)
Cabbage (35 calories)	½ cup reduced fat-feta cheese (140 calories)	1 Tbsp light Caesar (35 calories)
Kale (66 calories)	2 large eggs (156 calories)	1 Tbsp light mayonnaise (36 calories)
	3 oz grilled salmon (156 calories)	1 Tbsp light Italian (40 calories)
	2 1-oz slices reduced-fat cheese (160 calories)	

▶ Meal Component Swaps

Next, here are some charts to help you customize the meals you'll find in Chapters 5, 6, and 7. Or, pick one protein, one side dish, and one vegetable from the charts below to create your own lunch or dinner. Depending on what you pick and which phase you're in, you may also be able to add an item from the Fruit Swaps chart.

Again, you'll see that the foods in these charts cover a pretty wide calorie range, but all can fit into any phase of the diet, depending on how you combine them. If you're in Kickstart, stick with lower-calorie choices in all categories. In Steady Loss, you may want to balance out a higher-calorie protein with a lower-calorie side dish. In Maintain, you have free rein to pick whatever substitutions you like.

Protein Swaps (per 3 oz cooked unless otherwise indicated)

▶ Substitute any of these choices for protein in the meals

- Kidney beans, ½ cup (105 calories)
- Lentils, ½ cup (115 calories)
- Tofu, ⅔ cup (120 calories)
- Ground turkey (126 calories)
- 90% lean ground beef (132 calories)
- Skinless white meat chicken (140 calories)
- Chickpeas, ½ cup (143 calories)

- Tilapia, 4 oz (145 calories)
- Snapper, 4 oz (145 calories)
- Sirloin tip (150 calories)
- Top sirloin (156 calories)
- London broil (157 calories)
- Tri-tip (158 calories)
- Wild salmon, 4 oz (158 calories)
- Farmed salmon (174 calories)
- Bluefin tuna, 4 oz (209 calories)

Side Dish Swaps

▶ Substitute any of these choices for side dishes in the meals

- 1 cup home-roasted vegetables (100 calories)
- 1 medium baked potato or sweet potato (102 calories)
- ½ cup cooked brown rice (108 calories)
- ½ cup cooked pasta (110 calories)
- 1 cup Birds Eye Steamfresh Chef's Favorites Roasted Red Potatoes & Green Beans (120 calories)
- ⅔ cup prepared (from ⅓ box) Near East Tabouleh (120 calories)
- ½ cup Bush's Best Vegetarian Baked Beans (130 calories)

Vegetable Swaps

▶ **Substitute 1 cup of any of these choices for steamed or lightly sautéed vegetable in the meals**

- Zucchini (27 calories)
- Cabbage (34 calories)
- Mixed Asian vegetables (38 calories)
- Peppers (40 calories)
- Green beans (44 calories)
- Mushrooms (44 calories)
- Broccoli (55 calories)

Fruit Swaps

▶ **Substitute any of these choices for fruit in the meals**

- ½ cup strawberries (27 calories)
- ½ cup sliced peaches (30 calories)
- ½ cup raspberries (32 calories)
- ½ cup fresh blueberries (42 calories)
- ½ small banana (45 calories)
- ½ cup fruit salad (45 calories)
- ½ medium apple (48 calories)
- 1 small orange (50 calories)
- ½ grapefruit (52 calories)
- 2 Tbsp dried fruit (54 calories)
- 1 cup melon (55 calories)

Chapter 5
KICKSTART MEALS

Welcome to your Kickstart! Remember, this phase is designed to help you drop the pounds quickly. Every one of our 10 testers lost weight on this phase, most a pound a day or even more—Karen Woytach lost 10 pounds in 5 days! They all enjoyed newfound energy and had plenty of foods to choose from. Even though Kickstart is only 1200 calories per day, you still get a snack every day, you can still eat out if you choose, and you can still enjoy pizza, cheeseburgers, and chocolate.

Take a quick look at the menu to the right to see how a Kickstart day might compare to a sample pre-diet day.

You can see how following the Kickstart meals can help you drop a pound a day! The Kickstart meal plan gives you approximately 1200 calories per day, low enough to jump-start weight loss but high enough to allow for real food, real eating. Mindy has carefully planned your meals so that you can feel satisfied and get all the nutrition you need even at this calorie level. If, like most of us, you're used to eating much bigger portions of food, you might worry that you'll be hungry, but I encourage you to try the meals exactly as written. Your body will soon adjust to the smaller portions, and you'll be pleasantly surprised to find that you feel full even though you've eaten much less than you used to. As Eileen Supran reported, "At first, the food on the plan didn't look like it would be enough. But the recommended portions stopped me from overeating, and as my stomach got smaller, I felt the difference."

To get past your hunger pangs in the first few days, try the following strategies:

1) Break up one or two of your meals into smaller meals, so that you can eat more frequently. Karen Woytach reported, "I divided up breakfast and had part when I got up, part before going to the gym, and the last part when I finished. I felt GREAT and not hungry at all!"

SAMPLE PRE-DIET DAY

STOP EATING

BREAKFAST—Au Bon Pain

Eggs on a Bagel with Bacon and Cheese	**560 calories**
Medium Mocha Blast	**440 calories**
TOTAL	**1000 calories**

LUNCH—Home

Hamburger made with 1 Bubba Original Burger patty, on a kaiser roll with 2 slices American cheese	**774 calories**
½ cup potato salad	**162 calories**
½ cup deli coleslaw	**270 calories**
1 2-inch Ghirardelli Double Chocolate Brownie	**180 calories**
20-oz bottle soda	**240 calories**
TOTAL	**1626 calories**

DINNER—Home

Marie Callender's frozen Country Fried Chicken & Gravy with corn	**570 calories**
1 Pillsbury Grands! Flaky Layers Original Biscuits	**170 calories**
1 cup Rice-A-Roni Broccoli Au Gratin	**350 calories**
1 slice (⅛ pie) Edwards Key Lime Pie	**450 calories**
TOTAL	**1540 calories**

SNACK—Home

½ cup Lay's French Onion Dip	**240 calories**
28 (2 oz) Terra Chips	**300 calories**
2 12-oz bottles Sam Adams IPA	**350 calories**
TOTAL	**890 calories**

DAY TOTAL 5056 calories

SAMPLE KICKSTART DAY

START EATING

BREAKFAST—Home

1 slice Pepperidge Farm Whole Grain Honey Wheat Bread	**110 calories**
2 Mini Babybel Light cheeses	**100 calories**
1 medium apple	**94 calories**
TOTAL	**304 calories**

LUNCH—Wendy's

Jr. Cheeseburger	**280 calories**
Garden Side Salad, no croutons, with 1 Tbsp (½ packet) Light Honey French dressing	**45 calories**
Apple Slices	**35 calories**
Diet soda	**0 calories**
TOTAL	**360 calories**

DINNER—Home

Lean Cuisine Culinary Collection Herb Roasted Chicken	**180 calories**
2 cups baby lettuce or spring greens, plus chopped peppers, broccoli florets, and sprouts, sprinkled with vinegar and 4 quick sprays of olive oil	**25 calories**
2 Nabisco Oreo cookies	**106 calories**
1 cup fat-free milk	**80 calories**
TOTAL	**391 calories**

SNACK—Home

1.1 oz Popcorners Sea Salt Popped Corn Chips	**140 calories**
TOTAL	**140 calories**

DAY TOTAL 1195 calories

DROP: 3861 calories

2) Drink more water. Often, what you think is hunger is really thirst. Plus, water will help fill your tummy.

3) Go for a walk. This will distract you *and* help you burn a few calories.

4) Keep your goal in sight! Post a photo of yourself at a healthier weight or a motivational saying or even just your goal weight somewhere you'll see it regularly, and keep reminding yourself that you are worth it!

5) Remind yourself that this, too, shall pass. You'll only be staying at the 1200-calorie level for a week or so.

6) Munch on some raw green vegetables, such as celery, cucumbers, or bell peppers.

At this calorie level, you don't have a lot of wiggle room for foods that don't pack a lot of nutrition. So you'll see that almost all the meals and snacks in this chapter include several different components, including protein, grain, vegetables, and/or fruits. In this phase, it's especially important to measure all your food and stick as closely as you can to the products and dishes called for in the meal plan. Review the Stop & Drop FAQs in Chapter 4 closely so that you can avoid some of the challenges that our panelists ran across in this phase.

Kickstart at a Glance

Remember the fundamentals:

1. Choose one breakfast, one lunch, one dinner, and one snack per day. Lunches and dinners are interchangeable.

2. Eat meals approximately 4 hours apart. You can split any meal into two minimeals if you prefer to eat more frequently.

3. Follow the meal guidelines as closely as possible. If you do not consume dairy products, substitute calcium-fortified, unsweetened almond milk or light soy milk, or calcium-fortified juice for regular milk, and nondairy cheeses for cheese. If you are vegetarian, simply stick to the vegetarian options in the lists.

4. Walk an hour or more a day. You can break this into shorter walks, if needed.

5. Keep track of your eating, activity, and hunger levels on paper, on the computer, or with a phone app.

6. Take a multivitamin that provides 100% of the Daily Value for most vitamins and minerals (choose an iron-free formulation if you are a postmenopausal woman). Women should take a 600 mg calcium supplement daily.

If you pick from the Kickstart meals we've provided, every day you'll be getting approximately:

- 1200 calories
- 60 g of protein (include some at every meal and snack)
- 25 g of fiber
- 2400 mg of sodium
- 75 mg of vitamin C
- 1000 mg of calcium from a combination of foods (each dairy serving provides about 300 mg) and a supplement

To reach those nutritional goals, each day you should eat approximately:

- 4 ounces of grains and grain foods like breads and cereals, with at least half being whole grain
- 1½ cups of different kinds of veggies
- 1 cup of fruit
- 2 cups of milk or other calcium-rich beverages
- 4 ounces of protein foods

They will be spread out in your meals like so:

	Kickstart Meal Plan	Include These Types of Food
Breakfast	300 calories	Grain, fruit, dairy, and/or protein
Lunch & Dinner	350–400 calories	Vegetables, protein, grain, fruit, and/or dairy
Snack	1 x 150 calories	Fruit, vegetables, grain, and/or protein

Kickstart Breakfasts

Breakfast #1

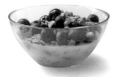

¾ cup Kellogg's All-Bran Original topped with ½ cup fresh blueberries, 1 Tbsp chopped walnuts, and 1 cup fat-free milk

293 calories

Breakfast #2

¾ cup Kashi GOLEAN Crunch!

1 cup fat-free milk

1 Tbsp raisins

300 calories

Breakfast #3

1 packet plain Quaker Instant Original Oatmeal topped with ½ cup chopped apple, 1 Tbsp shredded coconut, 1 Tbsp chopped pecans, and 1 tsp brown sugar

1 5.2–6 oz carton (80–100 calories) 0% plain Greek or light fat-free yogurt

299 calories

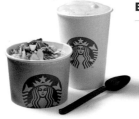

Breakfast #4

Starbucks Classic Whole-Grain Oatmeal topped with Starbucks Nut Medley

Starbucks Tall (12 oz) cappuccino or latte made with fat-free milk

320 calories

Breakfast #5

Kellogg's Special K Protein Almond Honey Oat Granola Bar

1 small banana

1 5.2–6 oz carton (80–100 calories) 0% plain Greek or light fat-free yogurt

290 calories

Breakfast #6

KIND Peanut Butter Dark Chocolate Healthy Grains bar

1 medium orange

1 5.2–6 oz carton (80–100 calories) 0% plain Greek or light fat-free yogurt

300 calories

Breakfast #7

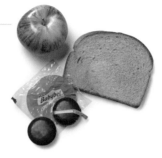

1 slice Pepperidge Farm Whole Grain Honey Wheat Bread

2 Mini Babybel Light cheeses

1 medium apple

304 calories

Breakfast #8

1 Thomas' Light Multi-Grain English Muffin with 1 Tbsp almond butter

1 5.3-oz carton Dannon Oikos Plain Nonfat Greek Yogurt with ½ cup raspberries

308 calories

Breakfast #9

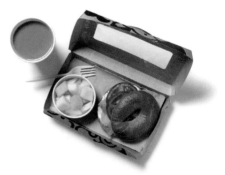

1 Einstein Bros. Bagels Honey Whole Wheat Bagel (ask for a "thin" bagel) with 1 Tbsp light cream cheese, 1 oz lox, 2 tomato slices

½ cup fruit salad

1 cup coffee with up to 4 Tbsp fat-free milk

308 calories

Breakfast #10

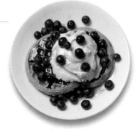

2 Kashi 7 Grain Waffles with 1 5.2–6 oz carton (80–100 calories) 0% plain Greek or light fat-free yogurt, ½ cup blueberries, and 2 tsp maple syrup

326 calories

Breakfast #11

Weight Watchers Smart Ones Three Cheese Omelet

½ grapefruit

½ cup fat-free milk

292 calories

Breakfast #12

1 Thomas' 100% Whole Wheat Bagel Thins bagel with 1 thin slice reduced-fat Swiss, 1 poached egg, and 1 tomato slice

1 medium orange

317 calories

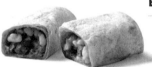

Breakfast #13

Good Food Made Simple Chicken Apple Sausage Egg White Breakfast Burrito

310 calories

Breakfast #14

Omelet made from 2 eggs, 1 egg white, 1 cup broccoli, 2 Tbsp Kraft Shredded Reduced Fat Mild Cheddar, and fresh herbs to taste in a nonstick pan coated with 2 sprays of cooking spray

1 slice Pepperidge Farm Very Thin 100% Whole Wheat Bread

293 calories

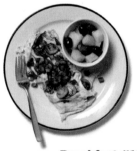

Breakfast #15

IHOP Simple & Fit Vegetable Omelette with fruit cup

320 calories

Breakfast #16

McDonald's Fruit 'n Yogurt Parfait

McDonald's Egg White Delight McMuffin (remove the top half of the muffin)

335 calories

Breakfast #17

1 5.3–oz carton Dannon Oikos Vanilla Nonfat Greek Yogurt

1 cup mixed berries

¼ cup Kellogg's Original Low Fat Granola

285 calories

Breakfast #18

2 slices Wasa Fiber Crispbread

Smoothie made with:

> 1 5.2–6 oz carton (80–100 calories) 0% plain Greek or light fat-free yogurt
>
> 1 Tbsp peanut butter
>
> 1 tsp honey
>
> ½ small apple, peeled, cored, and chopped
>
> Ice

305 calories

Breakfast #19

Smoothie made with:

> 1 cup frozen mixed berries
>
> ½ small banana, peeled and chopped
>
> 1 Tbsp almond butter
>
> 1 cup (60–80 calories) almond milk

287 calories

Breakfast #20

Juice made with:

> 1 cup kale, chopped
>
> 1 medium apple, peeled, cored, and chopped
>
> 1 medium carrot, peeled and chopped
>
> 1 mandarin orange, peeled
>
> 1 Tbsp almond or peanut butter
>
> 1-inch piece fresh ginger, peeled and chopped

289 calories

Kickstart Lunches

Lunch #1

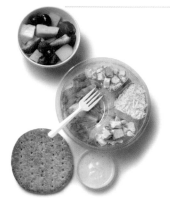

Ready Pac Bistro Bowl Caesar Lite Salad with chicken
(OR 2 cups romaine lettuce, 2 oz roasted chicken breast,
1 Tbsp shredded Parmesan cheese, and 1 Tbsp light
Caesar dressing)

1 Arnold 100% Whole Wheat Sandwich Thins roll

1 cup fruit salad

370 calories

Lunch #2

3 oz grilled salmon or chicken breast on top of 2 cups lettuce or mixed
greens with ¼ cup fresh herbs (basil, parsley, cilantro, dill), sprinkled with
lemon juice and 8 sprays of olive oil

1 Thomas' Light Multi-Grain English Muffin

373 calories

Lunch #3

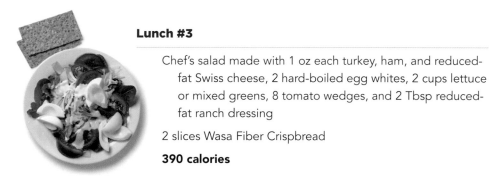

Chef's salad made with 1 oz each turkey, ham, and reduced-
fat Swiss cheese, 2 hard-boiled egg whites, 2 cups lettuce
or mixed greens, 8 tomato wedges, and 2 Tbsp reduced-
fat ranch dressing

2 slices Wasa Fiber Crispbread

390 calories

Lunch #4

1 pouch StarKist Albacore Ready-to-Eat Tuna Salad

1 hard-boiled egg

2 slices Wasa Fiber Crispbread

2 cups baby lettuce or spring greens plus chopped peppers, broccoli florets,
and sprouts, sprinkled with vinegar and 4 sprays of olive oil

½ cup grapes

347 calories

Lunch #5

McDonald's Premium Southwest Salad with Grilled Chicken with 1 packet Newman's Own Lite Balsamic Vinaigrette

330 calories

Lunch #6

Panera Greek Salad, with red vinegar

370 calories

Lunch #7

4 oz (5-oz can, drained) StarKist Chunk Light Tuna in Water with 1 Tbsp light mayo on 2 slices Pepperidge Farm Whole Grain Honey Wheat Bread, with lettuce and tomato

1 cup lettuce or mixed greens with tomatoes and cucumber, sprinkled with vinegar and 4 sprays of olive oil

380 calories

Lunch #8

2½ oz pretzel roll with 4 oz regular, smoked, or low-sodium turkey breast; lettuce, tomato, and mustard

½ cup (⅕ can) READ 3 Bean Salad

379 calories

Lunch #9

Baked open-face sandwich with 1 slice Pepperidge Farm Whole Grain Honey Wheat Bread, 3 Tbsp Kraft Shredded Reduced Fat Mild Cheddar, tomato slices, and roasted red peppers (place veggies and cheese on the bread and bake at 350°F)

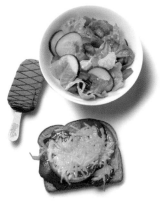

1 cup lettuce or mixed greens with tomatoes and cucumber, sprinkled with vinegar and 4 sprays of olive oil

Skinny Cow Chocolate Truffle Ice Cream Bar

370 calories

Lunch #10

Subway 6-inch Veggie Delite on 9-grain wheat bread

1 cup Subway Tomato Basil or Poblano Corn Chowder soup

370 calories

Lunch #11

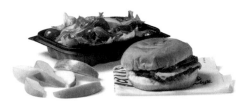

Wendy's Jr. Cheeseburger

Wendy's Garden Side Salad, no croutons, with 1 Tbsp
(½ packet) Light Honey French Dressing

Wendy's Apple Slices

370 calories

Lunch #12

1 cup (½ can) Amy's Organic Split Pea Soup

1 slice Pepperidge Farm Whole Grain Honey Wheat Bread

1-inch cube Cabot Sharp Light Cheddar

8 baby carrots

1 cup strawberries

364 calories

Lunch #13

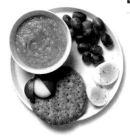

1 cup (½ can) Amy's Organic Split Pea Soup

1 Mini Babybel Light cheese

1 hard-boiled egg

1 Arnold 100% Whole Wheat Sandwich Thins roll

½ cup grapes

374 calories

Lunch #14

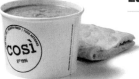

Regular Cosi Southwest Corn & Turkey Chili

½ piece Cosi Original Flatbread

397 calories

Lunch #15

Amy's Southwestern Burrito

1 cup fruit salad

380 calories

Lunch #16

Lean Cuisine Culinary Collection Baked Chicken

1 cup steamed broccoli

1 cup fruit salad

385 calories

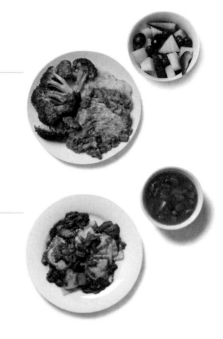

Lunch #17

Weight Watchers Smart Ones Ravioli Florentine

1 cup (½ can) Campbell's Chunky Savory
Vegetable Soup

370 calories

Lunch #18

1 5.3-oz carton Chobani Simply 100 Blueberry Greek Yogurt topped with
2 Tbsp chopped pecans, ¼ cup Nature's Path Fruit & Nut Granola, and
¼ cup blueberries

355 calories

Kickstart Dinners

Dinner #1

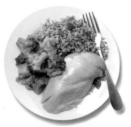

4 oz rotisserie chicken breast, no skin

⅔ cup prepared (from ⅓ box) Near East Tabouleh

½ cup Green Giant Steamers Broccoli & Cheese Sauce (measure out 1 cup—⅓ of a 12-oz bag—frozen broccoli from the bag; put the rest back in the freezer)

352 calories

Dinner #2

1 cup (½ can) Progresso Vegetable Classics Vegetarian Vegetable with Barley Soup

3 oz boneless, skinless chicken breast sautéed with 1 cup sliced mushrooms and ½ tsp olive oil in a nonstick pan

½ cup Uncle Ben's Ready Rice Whole Grain Brown Rice

352 calories

Dinner #3

Lean Cuisine Culinary Collection Herb Roasted Chicken

2 cups baby lettuce or spring greens plus chopped peppers, broccoli florets, and sprouts, sprinkled with vinegar and 4 sprays of olive oil

2 Nabisco Oreo cookies

1 cup fat-free milk

381 calories

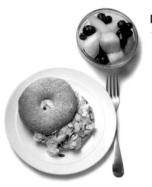

Dinner #4

Curry chicken salad made with 3 oz chopped chicken breast, 2 Tbsp plain 0% fat Greek yogurt, 1 Tbsp sliced almonds, and curry powder to taste on 1 Thomas' 100% Whole Wheat Bagel Thins bagel

1 cup fruit salad

390 calories

Dinner #5

Marie Callender's Chicken Pot Pie (remove the top crust) (restaurant entrée)

Marie Callender's Spring Side Salad with pecans, mandarin oranges, and vinegar (no craisins or dressing)

410 calories

Dinner #6

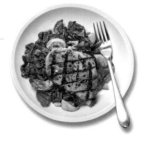

TGI Friday's Sizzling Chicken and Spinach (restaurant entrée)

410 calories

Dinner #7

1 cup (½ can) Progresso Traditional Manhattan Clam Chowder

6 oz baked tilapia, sprinkled with fresh herbs

1 cup steamed broccoli

373 calories

Dinner #8

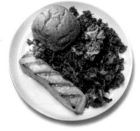

4 oz grilled salmon

2 cups fresh greens of your choice (kale, spinach, chard, bok choy, etc.) and 1 tsp chopped garlic (optional), sautéed with ½ tsp oil in a nonstick pan

1 small whole wheat roll

367 calories

Dinner #9

1 cup miso soup

1 tuna avocado roll (6 pieces) and 1 spicy salmon roll (6 pieces)

1 cup green salad with 1 Tbsp carrot-ginger salad dressing

393 calories

Dinner #10

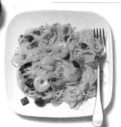

Lean Cuisine Culinary Collection Shrimp and Angel Hair Pasta

Skinny Cow Vanilla Ice Cream Sandwich

380 calories

Dinner #11

3 oz lean roast beef

1 medium baked sweet potato

2 cups fresh greens of your choice (kale, spinach, chard, bok choy, etc.) and 1 tsp chopped garlic (optional), sautéed in ½ tsp oil in a nonstick pan

½ cup cantaloupe cubes

369 calories

Dinner #12

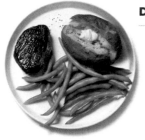

3 oz top sirloin steak

Medium baked potato with 1 tsp I Can't Believe It's Not Butter

1 cup steamed green beans

391 calories

Dinner #13

Chili's Lighter Choice 6 oz Classic Sirloin

Chili's House Salad, no dressing, with vinegar

390 calories

Dinner #14

⅓ order Chili's Fresh Mex Fajitas with Grilled Steak, peppers, onions, and toppings

1 tortilla

1 order Chili's avocado slices

407 calories

Dinner #15

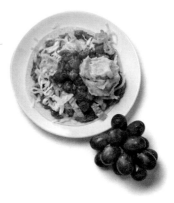

Corn tortilla topped with ½ cup Old El Paso Black Bean Refried Beans, 2 Tbsp Wholly Guacamole Classic, ¼ cup Santa Barbara Garden Style Salsa, 2 Tbsp Sargento Shredded Reduced Fat 4 Cheese Mexican cheese, and shredded lettuce

½ cup grapes

334 calories

Dinner #16

1 Boca All American Flame Grilled Veggie Burger on a whole wheat hamburger bun with lettuce, tomato, and ketchup

½ cup Bush's Best Vegetarian Baked Beans

393 calories

Dinner #17

Amy's Vegetable Lasagna

370 calories

Dinner #18

CedarLane Eggplant Parmesan

1 cup lettuce or mixed greens with tomatoes and cucumber, sprinkled with vinegar and 4 sprays of olive oil

1 cup cantaloupe cubes

364 calories

Dinner #19

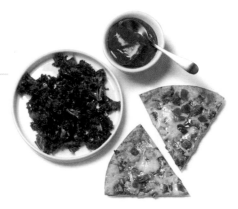

⅓ Kashi Thin Crust Pizza Margherita

1 cup fresh greens of your choice (kale, spinach, chard, bok choy, etc.) and 1 tsp chopped garlic (optional), sautéed in ½ tsp oil in a nonstick pan

½ cup prepared Royal Instant Sugar Free Reduced Calorie Pudding, made with fat-free milk

390 calories

Kickstart Snacks

Snack #1

1 cup fruit salad with 1 Tbsp chopped walnuts

138 calories

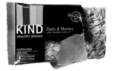

Snack #2

1 small banana with 2 tsp peanut butter

150 calories

Snack #3

21 roasted almonds

146 calories

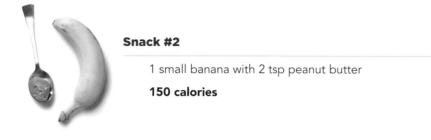

Snack #4

KIND Oats & Honey with Toasted Coconut bar

150 calories

Snack #5

1 5.3-oz carton Chobani Blended Lemon Greek Yogurt

130 calories

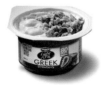

Snack #6

1 5.3-oz carton Dannon Light & Fit Greek Nonfat Strawberry Yogurt topped with 2 Tbsp Nature's Path Granola, any flavor

150 calories

Snack #7

½ Arnold 100% Whole Wheat Sandwich Thins roll topped with 2 tsp peanut butter

½ medium apple, sliced

159 calories

Snack #8

¼ cup Athenos Roasted Red Pepper Hummus

10 baby carrots

5 cherry tomatoes

150 calories

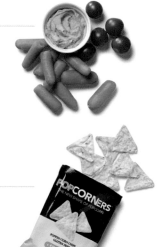

Snack #9

1.1 oz Popcorners Sea Salt Popped Corn Chips

140 calories

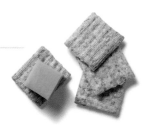

Snack #10

2 Tbsp Classic Wholly Guacamole

10 Snyder's of Hanover Mini Pretzels

165 calories

Snack #11

1-inch cube Cabot Sharp Light Cheddar Cheese

4 Reduced Fat Triscuit crackers

143 calories

Snack #12

8 large shrimp in ¼ cup cocktail sauce

1 slice Wasa Fiber Crispbread

155 calories

Snack #13

Panda Express Chicken Potstickers

160 calories

Snack #14

1 container Campbell's Soup on the Go Classic Tomato Soup

140 calories

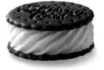

Snack #15

Skinny Cow Vanilla Ice Cream Sandwich

150 calories

Snack #16

Fruttare Strawberry Bar

4 Hershey's Special Dark Kisses

144 calories

Snack #17

3 Keebler Fudge Shoppe Cheesecake Middles Original Graham cookies

130 calories

Snack #18

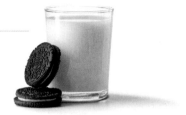

2 Nabisco Oreos

¾ cup fat-free milk

156 calories

Chapter 6
STEADY LOSS MEALS

I hope the Kickstart phase was as exciting for you as it was for our testers! By now, you should be accustomed to eating small, balanced meals and snacks throughout the day. But as I cautioned, Kickstart is designed to be just that: a short burst to get you going and boost your motivation. Now it's time to settle into a diet that you can follow in the weeks and months to come as you work toward reaching your weight loss goal.

The menu at right shows you what a difference a few simple changes can make.

The biggest difference between this phase and the Kickstart meals is, of course, the calories. I've added around 400 daily calories by giving you slightly bigger meals plus an extra snack. More food and more variety will make it easier to get the nutrients you need on a daily basis.

Your weight loss may slow down in this phase. But even though you're increasing your calorie consumption, you can still keep the pounds coming off. Here are a few strategies you can use to break through a plateau:

1) Stick with it! When the scale doesn't budge, you may be tempted to cut calories even more. That can backfire, as your body may react to the diet by trying to hang on to its stored fat. Have patience, stick with the Steady Loss meals (maybe mixing in a Kickstart meal or two), and trust that you will lose weight again soon enough.

2) Keep moving. Exercise can help you break through a plateau by boosting your metabolism and increasing your muscle mass, which burns more calories at rest than fat does. In addition to walking, try weight training or other weight-bearing activities to build muscle.

3) Spot-check your habits. Even after just a week or two of dieting, it can be easy to slide back into old habits. Reread the list of top diet saboteurs in Chapter 1 to make sure you haven't fallen prey to any of them. Remember to stop and think before you eat so that you can make smart choices.

SAMPLE PRE-DIET DAY		SAMPLE STEADY LOSS DAY	
STOP EATING		**START EATING**	
BREAKFAST—Home		**BREAKFAST—Home**	
3 scrambled eggs with 1 slice cheddar cheese	387 calories	2 scrambled eggs with 1 tsp olive oil	182 calories
Alvarado St. Bakery Sprouted Wheat Bagel, with 2 Tbsp cream cheese	359 calories	1 Thomas' Light Multi-Grain English Muffin	100 calories
Coffee with 2 Tbsp half-and-half	39 calories	8 oz latte made with cup each hot fat-free milk and coffee	50 calories
TOTAL	**785 calories**	**TOTAL**	**332 calories**
LUNCH—Chipotle		**LUNCH—Chipotle**	
Burrito Bowl with carnitas, brown rice, pinto beans, fajita vegetables, tomatillo green chili salsa, sour cream, cheese and lettuce, plus a side of chips and guacamole	1585 calories	Chipotle salad made with barbacoa, brown rice, fajita vegetables, fresh tomato salsa, lettuce	415 calories
TOTAL	**1585 calories**	**TOTAL**	**415 calories**
DINNER—Longhorn Steakhouse		**DINNER—Home**	
8 oz Prime Rib Steak	520 calories	3 oz London broil	157 calories
Caesar Side Salad with Caesar Dressing	280 calories	1 cup Idahoan Au Gratin Homestyle Casserole	150 calories
Loaded Baked Potato	440 calories	½ cup sautéed spinach	30 calories
¼ of an Caramel Apple Goldrush	410 calories	6 oz glass Pinot Grigio	125 calories
Ultimate Steakhouse Martini	220 calories		
TOTAL	**1870 calories**	**TOTAL**	**462 calories**
SNACK—Home		**SNACK—Home**	
½ cup Talenti Double Dark Chocolate Gelato	210 calories	½ cup Breyers Triple Chocolate Gelato Indulgences	160 calories
		2 Nabisco Nilla Wafers	35 calories
TOTAL	**210 calories**	**TOTAL**	**195 calories**
SNACK—Home		**SNACK—Home**	
1 block Nissin Top Ramen Chicken Flavor	380 calories	1 container The Spice Hunter Reduced Sodium Split Pea Vegetarian Soup Cup	190 calories
TOTAL	**380 calories**	**TOTAL**	**190 calories**
DAY TOTAL 4830 calories		**DAY TOTAL 1594 calories**	

DROP: 3236 calories

4) Analyze your food journal. You should have been tracking what you eat, how you feel, and what exercise you do. Reread your journal for the past few days to see if you can spot any patterns that may be getting in the way of your weight loss. Maybe you always get busy in the late afternoon as you try to wrap up your day, so you go more than 6 hours between lunch and dinner and forget to measure your portions at dinner. Maybe you like to snuggle with your spouse after you get the kids to bed, and sneak in an extra spoonful or two of his ice cream while you relax.

5) Measure everything. You may think you've figured out what proper portions are in the Kickstart phase, but remember that you're getting slightly larger portions in the Steady Loss phase. You want to make sure you get enough to satisfy you but not so much more that you accidentally end up with Maintain-level calories. So keep the food scale and measuring cups handy!

At this calorie level, you have a little more room to enjoy snacks, desserts, and drinks. In fact, on this phase, I encourage you to add a second snack to make sure you don't get hungry between meals. This made our testers very happy, and I hope it makes you happy, too! But you still want to maximize nutrition, so you'll see that most of the meals and snacks are composed of several different food groups, including protein, grain, vegetables, and/or fruits. In this phase, you can do more mixing and matching to allow for more variety in your meals, but it's still important to keep a close eye on your portions.

Steady Loss at a Glance

Remember the fundamentals:

1. Choose one breakfast, one lunch, one dinner, and two snacks per day. Lunches and dinners are interchangeable.

2. Eat meals approximately 4 hours apart. You can split any meal into two minimeals if you prefer to eat more frequently.

3. Follow the meal guidelines as closely as possible. If you do not consume dairy products, substitute calcium-fortified, unsweetened almond milk or light soy milk, or calcium-fortified juice for regular milk, and nondairy cheeses for cheese. If you are vegetarian, simply stick to the vegetarian options in the lists.

4. Walk an hour or more a day. You can break this into shorter walks, if needed.

5. Keep track of your eating, activity, and hunger levels on paper, on the computer, or with a phone app.

6. Take a multivitamin that provides 100% of the Daily Value for most vitamins and minerals (choose an iron-free formulation if you are a postmenopausal woman). Women should take a 600 mg calcium supplement daily.

If you pick from the Steady Loss meals we've provided, you'll be getting approximately:

- 1600 calories
- 60 g of protein (include some at every meal and snack)
- 25 g of fiber
- 2400 mg of sodium
- 75 mg of vitamin C
- 1000 mg of calcium from a combination of foods (each dairy serving provides about 300 mg) and a supplement

To reach those daily nutritional goals, each day you should eat approximately:

- 5 ounces of grains and grain foods like breads and cereals, with at least half being whole grain
- 2 cups of different kinds of veggies
- 1½ cups of fruit
- 3 cups of milk or other calcium-rich beverages
- 5 ounces of protein foods

They will be spread out in your meals like so:

	Steady Loss Meal Plan	Include These Types of Food
Breakfast	350 calories	Grain, fruit, dairy, and/or protein
Lunch & Dinner	400–450 calories	Vegetables, protein, grain, fruit, and/or dairy
Snack	2 x 200 calories	Fruit, vegetables, grain, and/or protein

Steady Loss Breakfasts

Breakfast #1

¾ cup Wheat Chex topped with 1 small banana, 2 Tbsp sliced almonds, and
  ½ cup fat-free milk

358 calories

Breakfast #2

¾ cup Nature's Path Flax Plus Flakes, topped with 2 Tbsp chopped pecans,
  1 sliced peach, and 1 cup fat-free milk

344 calories

Breakfast #3

¾ cup Kashi GOLEAN Crunch! layered with 1 5.3-oz carton
  Dannon Oikos Plain Nonfat Greek Yogurt and 1 small
  cubed pear

354 calories

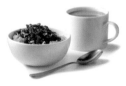

Breakfast #4

1 cup (½ box) Good Food Made Simple Steel Cut Oats
  Oatmeal topped with 2 Tbsp chopped pecans and 2 Tbsp
  raisins

8 oz latte made with ½ cup each hot fat-free milk and coffee

343 calories

Breakfast #5

2 slices toasted Pepperidge Farm Whole Grain Honey Wheat Bread topped
  with 1 Tbsp peanut or almond butter

½ medium apple, sliced

362 calories

Breakfast #6

2 Van's 8 Whole Grains Pancakes topped with 1 5.3-oz carton Chobani Fruit on the Bottom Strawberry Banana Greek Yogurt and ½ cup sliced strawberries

337 calories

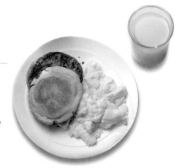

Breakfast #7

1 Thomas' Light Multi-Grain English Muffin topped with ¼ cup part-skim ricotta (with vanilla and noncaloric sweetener if desired)

1 cup fruit salad

1 cup fat-free milk

356 calories

Breakfast #8

2 eggs scrambled with 1 tsp olive oil or butter

1 Thomas' Light Multi-Grain English Muffin

1 cup Trop50 No Pulp Calcium + Vitamin D orange juice

332 calories

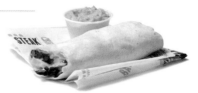

Breakfast #9

Good Food Made Simple Turkey Sausage Breakfast Burrito

½ grapefruit

352 calories

Breakfast #10

Taco Bell Cheesy Steak and Egg Fresco Style Burrito

Side order Taco Bell guacamole

355 calories

Breakfast #11

Starbucks Spinach & Feta Breakfast Wrap

Starbucks Seasonal Harvest Fruit Blend

380 calories

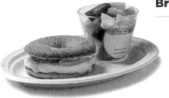

Breakfast #12

Au Bon Pain Egg Whites, Cheddar & Avocado on
a Skinny Wheat Bagel

Au Bon Pain Fruit Cup

380 calories

Breakfast #13

IHOP Simple & Fit Vegetable Omelette with fruit cup

1 cup coffee with up to 4 Tbsp fat-free milk

340 calories

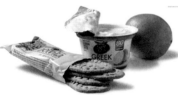

Breakfast #14

4 (1 package) belVita Golden Oat crunchy Breakfast Biscuits

1 medium orange

1 5.3-oz carton Dannon Light & Fit Greek Yogurt, any flavor

379 calories

Breakfast #15

KIND Vanilla Blueberry Healthy Grains bar

1 small banana

1 5.3-oz carton Dannon Oikos Plain Nonfat Greek Yogurt with 1 tsp honey

331 calories

Breakfast #16

Starbucks Greek Yogurt with Berries Parfait

Quaker Chewy Chocolate Chip Granola Bar

1 cup coffee with with up to 4 Tbsp fat-free milk

340 calories

Breakfast #17

Stonyfield Organic Strawberry Banana Smoothie

1 muffin made from Fiber One Blueberry Muffin mix

390 calories

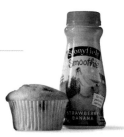

Steady Loss Lunches

Lunch #1

Ready Pac Bistro Bowl Asian Style Chicken Salad

1 5.3-oz carton Dannon Oikos Plain Nonfat Greek Yogurt

1 cup fruit salad with 1 Tbsp chopped nuts, any kind

430 calories

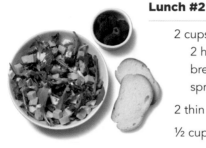

Lunch #2

2 cups mixed greens or baby romaine lettuce topped with 2 hard-boiled egg whites, ½ cup diced smoked chicken breast, and ¼ cup each diced tomato and avocado, sprinkled with vinegar and 4 sprays of olive oil

2 thin slices Italian bread

½ cup raspberries

425 calories

Lunch #3

½ cup cooked quinoa, ½ cup black beans, 2 Tbsp sliced almonds, and 1½ cups Cut'N Clean Greens SuperKALE Salad Slaw or other kale or greens salad mix, sprinkled with vinegar and 4 sprays of olive oil

1 small whole wheat roll

438 calories

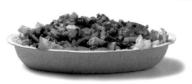

Lunch #4

Chipotle salad made with barbacoa, brown rice, fajita vegetables, fresh tomato salsa, lettuce, and tomato

415 calories

Lunch #5

TGI Friday's lunch menu Grilled Chicken Cobb Salad with Caesar Vinaigrette

400 calories

Lunch #6

2 slices whole wheat bread with 4 oz sliced turkey breast, 1 tsp deli mustard, lettuce, and tomato

½ cup no-mayo coleslaw or pickled vegetables

1 medium apple

454 calories

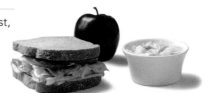

Lunch #7

2 slices Pepperidge Farm Whole Grain Honey Wheat Bread with 4 tsp peanut butter, 2 tsp all-fruit jam, and ¼ cup banana slices

8 oz latte made with ½ cup each hot fat-free milk and coffee

435 calories

Lunch #8

Burger King Double Hamburger

Burger King Side Garden Salad with 2 Tbsp (½ packet) Lite Honey Balsamic dressing

450 calories

Lunch #9

McDonald's Grilled Sweet Chili Chicken Premium McWrap

McDonald's Cuties

420 calories

Lunch #10

Subway 6-inch Sweet Onion Chicken Teriyaki Sandwich on 9-grain wheat bread

Subway Veggie Delite Salad with 1½ Tbsp fat-free vinaigrette (ask for dressing on the side)

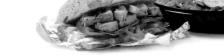

450 calories

Lunch #11

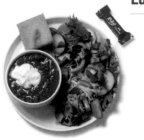

1 cup (½ can) Hormel Turkey Chili No Beans topped with 2 Tbsp plain 0% Greek yogurt

2 cups lettuce or mixed greens with tomato, cucumber, and peppers, sprinkled with vinegar and 8 sprays of olive oil

2-inch-square cornbread or 1 mini corn muffin

1 KitKat Miniature wafer

423 calories

Lunch #12

1 cup (½ can) Campbell's Healthy Request New England Clam Chowder

Tuna sandwich with 2½ oz chunk light tuna in water and 1 Tbsp light mayo on 2 slices Pepperidge Farm Very Thin 100% Whole Wheat Bread

1 cup lettuce or mixed greens with tomatoes and cucumber, sprinkled with vinegar and 4 sprays of olive oil

½ cup grapes

396 calories

Lunch #13

1 cup Pacific Organic Butternut Squash Bisque

Amy's Light & Lean Spaghetti Italiano Bowl

1 Snack Pack Fat Free Tapioca Pudding

430 calories

Lunch #14

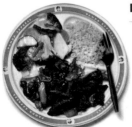

Panda Express kids' meal Shanghai Angus Steak

Panda Express kids' meal 6.4 oz Mixed Veggies side

⅓ order (⅓ cup) Panda Express kids' meal Brown Steamed Rice

413 calories

Lunch #15

1 cup Chili's Southwest Chicken Soup (Southwest Pairings menu)

1 Chili's Chicken Soft Taco (Southwest Pairings menu)

Chili's House Salad, no dressing, with vinegar or salsa

440 calories

Lunch #16

Lean Cuisine Comfort Meatloaf
   with Mashed Potatoes

½ bag Dole Light Caesar Salad Kit

Chobani Simply 100 Greek Yogurt, any flavor

430 calories

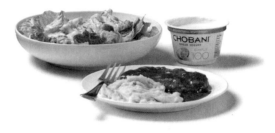

Lunch #17

Weight Watchers Smart Ones Chicken Oriental

1 medium orange

Nature Valley Oats 'n Honey Crunchy Granola Bar

409 calories

Lunch #18

⅓ of a Newman's Own Uncured Pepperoni Thin & Crispy
   Crust Pizza

1 cup lettuce or mixed greens with tomatoes and
   cucumber, sprinkled with vinegar and 4 sprays of
   olive oil

350 calories

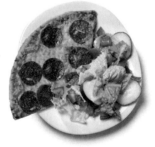

Lunch #19

Starbucks Protein Bistro Box

Starbucks Seasonal Harvest Fruit Blend

470 calories

Steady Loss Dinners

Dinner #1

4 oz boneless, skinless chicken breast stir-fried with 2 cups frozen or 1 cup fresh mixed Asian vegetables in 1 tsp oil in a nonstick pan (season with soy sauce)

¾ cup cooked brown rice

1 clementine orange

431 calories

Dinner #2

4 oz grilled boneless, skinless chicken breast

½ cup cooked quinoa

1 cup steamed broccoli

½ cup fruit salad

398 calories

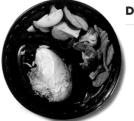

Dinner #3

Boston Market Quarter White Rotisserie Chicken, skinless

Boston Market Fresh Steamed Vegetables

Boston Market Garlic Dill New Potatoes

400 calories

Dinner #4

Banquet Turkey Meal

1 cup Dole or other coleslaw mix tossed with vinegar, a pinch of salt, and noncaloric sweetener to taste

Blueberry crumble made with 1 cup blueberries and a topping of 1 Tbsp each oats and sliced almonds, ½ tsp butter, 1 tsp sugar, and ¼ tsp cinnamon, baked at 350°F until lightly browned

438 calories

Dinner #5

Olive Garden Lasagna Primavera with Grilled Chicken

470 calories

Dinner #6

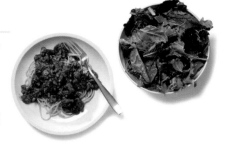

½ cup cooked Barilla ProteinPLUS spaghetti with ½ cup each cooked 93% lean ground turkey and Barilla Traditional Sauce

½ package Earthbound Farm Organic Garden Party Salad, sprinkled with vinegar and 4 sprays of olive oil (do not use dressing that comes with the package)

431 calories

Dinner #7

1 bowl Evol Butternut Squash and Sage Ravioli

1 cup (½ can) Wolfgang Puck Organic Classic Minestrone

440 calories

Dinner #8

Michelina's Lean Gourmet Shrimp with Pasta and Vegetables

1 cup cantaloupe cubes

15 almonds

398 calories

Dinner #9

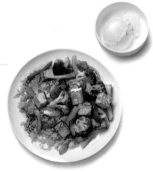

Stir-fry made with ½ cup cubed firm tofu, 2 cups fresh or 1½ cups frozen assorted stir-fry vegetables (no sauce or seasoning), 1 tsp oil, and 1 Tbsp teriyaki sauce

½ cup cooked brown rice

½ cup fat-free vanilla frozen yogurt

399 calories

Dinner #10

4 oz grilled salmon with 2 Tbsp teriyaki sauce

½ cup cooked brown rice

1 cup sautéed mixed vegetables

Nestlé Outshine Fruit Bar, No Sugar Added, any flavor

420 calories

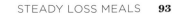

Dinner #11

Red Lobster Oven-Broiled Flounder

½ order Red Lobster Wild Rice Pilaf

Red Lobster Broccoli

435 calories

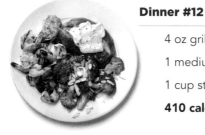

Dinner #12

4 oz grilled shrimp

1 medium baked potato with 2 Tbsp 0% plain Greek yogurt

1 cup steamed broccoli topped with 1 Tbsp sliced almonds

410 calories

Dinner #13

Red Lobster Create Your Own Combination portion Garlic-Grilled Shrimp

½ order Red Lobster Mashed Potatoes

Red Lobster Petite Green Beans

420 calories

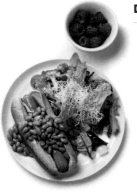

Dinner #14

1 Oscar Mayer Bun-Length Turkey Frank in 1 whole wheat hot dog bun

½ cup (½ of 8.3-oz can) Bush's Best Vegetarian Baked Beans

2 cups baby lettuce or spring greens plus chopped peppers, broccoli florets, and sprouts, sprinkled with vinegar and 4 sprays of olive oil

½ cup raspberries

423 calories

Dinner #15

3 oz London broil

1 cup Idahoan Au Gratin Homestyle Casserole

½ cup spinach, sautéed with 1 tsp olive oil in a nonstick pan

6 oz glass Pinot Grigio

462 calories

Dinner #16

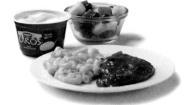

Lean Cuisine Culinary Collection Salisbury Steak with
Macaroni & Cheese

1 5.3-oz carton Dannon Oikos Plain Nonfat Greek Yogurt

1 cup fruit salad

430 calories

Dinner #17

Panda Express Broccoli Beef with ½ order steamed brown rice

430 calories

Dinner #18

6 oz Outback Steakhouse Special Sirloin

Outback Fresh Steamed Broccoli

391 calories

Dinner #19

Lean Cuisine Simple Favorites French Bread Cheese Pizza

2 cups baby lettuce or spring greens plus chopped peppers, broccoli florets,
and sprouts, sprinkled with vinegar and 4 sprays of olive oil

1 cup cantaloupe cubes

435 calories

Dinner #20

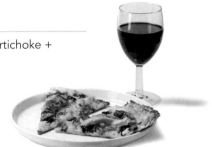

¼ of a California Pizza Kitchen Roasted Artichoke +
Spinach with Chicken pizza

6 oz glass European red wine
(ABV 11–13.5%)

457 calories

Steady Loss Snacks

Snack #1

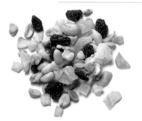

⅓ cup homemade or packaged fruit and nut trail mix

210 calories

Snack #2

1 oz (about 9) chocolate-covered almonds

1 Tbsp dried cherries

194 calories

Snack #3

KIND Healthy Grains bar, any flavor

2 Tbsp raisins

204 calories

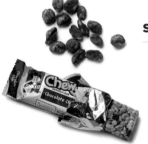

Snack #4

Quaker Chewy Chocolate Chip Granola Bar

1 Tbsp Planters Cocoa Peanuts

180 calories

Snack #5

1 cup fruit salad

1 5.3-oz carton Chobani Simply 100 Greek Yogurt, any flavor

190 calories

Snack #6

2 Mini Babybel Light cheeses

4-inch (1 oz) whole wheat pita, split into two halves, sprayed with 4 sprays of oil, each cut into 4 wedges and baked at 350°F until crisp

214 calories

Snack #7

¼ cup Tribe Classic Hummus

4-inch (1 oz) whole wheat pita

8 baby carrots

212 calories

Snack #8

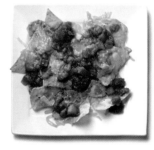

9 tortilla chips topped with 3 Tbsp each fat-free refried beans, shredded reduced-fat cheddar cheese, and salsa

215 calories

Snack #9

61 (1 oz) EatSmart Garden Veggie Straws

2 Tbsp Sabra Cucumber Dill Greek Yogurt Dip

170 calories

Snack #10

1 medium baked sweet potato topped with ¼ cup Sabra Cucumber Dill Greek Yogurt Dip

182 calories

Snack #11

1 container The Spice Hunter Reduced Sodium Split Pea Vegetarian Soup Cup

190 calories

Snack #12

1 container Campbell's Soup on the Go Classic Tomato soup

3 Reduced Fat Triscuit crackers

195 calories

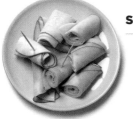

Snack #13

Roll-ups made with 3 slices (3 oz) low-sodium deli turkey breast and 2 thin slices (about 1¼ oz) reduced-fat provolone

180 calories

Snack #14

3 pieces Tyson Buffalo Style Boneless Chicken Wyngz

1 Tbsp ketchup

169 calories

Snack #15

3 Mrs. T's Savory Onion Pierogies

160 calories

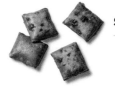

Snack #16

1 pouch (½ package) Lean Cuisine Monterey Jack Jalapeño Stuffed Pretzels

190 calories

Snack #17

2 Trader Joe's Soft Bite Mini Almond Biscotti

12 oz latte made with ¾ cup each hot fat-free milk and coffee

200 calories

Snack #18

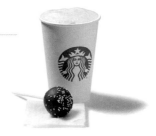

Starbucks Chocolate Cake Pop

Starbucks Tall (12 oz) nonfat cappuccino

200 calories

Snack #19

½ cup Breyers Triple Chocolate Gelato Indulgences

2 Nabisco Nilla Wafers

195 calories

Snack #20

Klondike No Sugar Added Krunch bar

170 calories

Snack #21

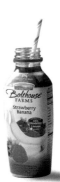

1 15.2-oz bottle Bolthouse Farms Strawberry Banana
Smoothie

230 calories

Snack #22

16 oz Jamba Juice Strawberries Wild Make It Light Smoothie

8 Popchips Sea Salt Potato Chips (⅓ of a 1-oz bag)

200 calories

Chapter 7
MAINTAIN MEALS

Congratulations! You've made it to Maintain, where your new goal is to hold on to your hard-earned weight loss rather than shedding more pounds. You might be surprised to hear me say this, but while anyone can lose weight, most of us are much better at gaining it back. We take our eye off the ball. Once we've reached our goal weight, we relax and pay less attention to our choices and our portions. The little things add up—whole milk instead of fat free, 2 slices of toast instead of one, a creamy pasta salad instead of a vegetable salad, nachos instead of chips and salsa. We're talking 20 calories here, 100 calories there. Over the course of a week or month, the surplus adds up. Our pants get tighter, the number on the scale creeps up, and we're back where we started.

See the example at right of how making just a few less-than-healthy choices can lead to a big calorie difference over the course of a day.

But guess what? You CAN keep the weight off by continuing to do what you've been doing for the past weeks: Stop eating calorie-rich, nutrition-poor foods that pack on the pounds and start eating meals and snacks that are smart, have the right number of calories, and fit into your lifestyle.

The Maintain meals and snacks here add up to approximately 2000 calories per day. This matches the government's recommendations for daily calories for an average adult. With this generous number of calories, it's pretty easy to meet your nutrition needs and enjoy a wide variety of foods.

You may find that the scale starts going up when you switch to the Maintain phase. That means you're not exactly an average adult; your sweet spot for daily calories may lie somewhere between 1600 and 2000. So mix and match between the Steady Loss and Maintain meals, and even hold on to some of your favorite Kickstart meals, until you find a combination that keeps your weight steady. You may find that your weight stays steady at the Steady Loss level, which is also perfectly normal. If that's the case, feel free to stay at the Steady Loss phase indefinitely and just use the Maintain meals to help you make smart choices for the occasional treat.

SAMPLE RELAXED DIET DAY | SAMPLE MAINTAIN DAY

STOP EATING		START EATING	
BREAKFAST—Home		**BREAKFAST—Home**	
⅔ cup Cascadian Farm Fruit and Nut Granola cereal	230 calories	½ cup Kellogg's Frosted Mini Wheats	190 calories
1 cup whole milk	150 calories	1 medium banana	106 calories
1 Jiffy corn muffin (from mix)	170 calories	1½ Tbsp walnuts	72 calories
		1 cup fat-free milk	83 calories
TOTAL	550 calories	**TOTAL**	451 calories
LUNCH—Sonic		**LUNCH—Panera**	
Grilled Cheese Sandwich	410 calories	½ Classic Grilled Cheese	290 calories
Small Vanilla Shake	540 calories	½ Greek Salad with 1½ Tbsp (½ portion) Panera Reduced Fat Balsamic Vinaigrette	250 calories
TOTAL	950 calories	**TOTAL**	540 calories
DINNER—Bertucci's		**DINNER—Bonefish Grill**	
1 Maryland Style Crab Cake	550 calories	Small order Chilean Sea Bass	345 calories
Small Caesar Salad	260 calories	½ order Herbed Couscous	148 calories
Grilled Salmon	680 calories	Steamed Asparagus	44 calories
Broccoli side	310 calories		
TOTAL	1800 calories	**TOTAL**	537 calories
SNACK—Home		**SNACK—Home**	
Haagen Dazs Vanilla Milk Chocolate Almond Ice Cream Bar	300 calories	Red Mango 16 oz Strawberry-Banana Fruit & Yogurt Smoothie	240 calories
TOTAL	300 calories	**TOTAL**	240 calories
SNACK—Taco Bell		**SNACK—Home**	
Chips and Nacho Cheese Sauce	310 calories	½ cup (¼ recipe) salsa made with 1 chopped medium tomato, 1 chopped avocado, 2 Tbsp minced onion, juice of ½ lime, salt to taste, and chopped jalapeño and cilantro if desired	90 calories
		10 (1 oz) Food Should Taste Good Multigrain Tortilla Chips	140 calories
TOTAL	310 calories	**TOTAL**	230 calories
DAY TOTAL 3910 calories		**DAY TOTAL 1998 calories**	

DROP: 1912 calories

You will see that in this phase I've included a few meals and snacks that are no one's idea of health food (pretzels, chips, cake). That's because this phase is designed to take you through the rest of your life. Hey, there's no reason for anyone to go the rest of their life without cake! While all the meals and snacks in this chapter include real food that real people eat, not all are perfectly balanced on their own. So mix and match meals from this chapter to meet the suggested food goals. I think you'll find plenty to choose from!

I've packed this book with lots of tools—foods to stop and start, sample meals, swap charts—to help you make smart choices in your daily food decisions. Mindy and I put together lots of examples of different types of meals and snacks, including pure splurges like candy and ice cream, to show you that nearly everything can fit within the framework of a healthy diet.

I've found that eating in a consistent way is the key to keeping my weight where I want it. As soon as I stray too far by eating the wrong foods or slacking off in my exercise, I feel my jeans tighten and see my face fill out. That's my reminder to get back on track. I know that you can also succeed at stopping your bad habits, starting to eat smart, dropping all the weight you want . . . and keeping it off!

Maintain at a Glance

Remember the fundamentals (note that in this phase, you're getting enough calories that you can meet all your nutritional needs without taking a multivitamin; you may still want to take one for added insurance anyway!):

1. Choose one breakfast, one lunch, one dinner, and two snacks per day. Lunches and dinners are interchangeable.

2. Eat meals approximately 4 hours apart. You can split any meal into two minimeals if you prefer to eat more frequently.

3. Follow the meal guidelines as closely as possible. If you do not consume dairy products, substitute calcium-fortified, unsweetened almond milk or light soy milk, or calcium-fortified juice for regular milk, and nondairy cheeses for cheese. If you are vegetarian, simply stick to the vegetarian options in the lists.

4. Walk an hour or more a day. You can break this into shorter walks, if needed.

5. Keep track of your eating, activity, and hunger levels on paper, on the computer, or with a phone app.

If you pick from the Maintain meals we've provided, you'll be getting approximately:

- 2000 calories
- 60 g of protein (include some at every meal and snack)
- 25 g of fiber
- 2400 mg of sodium
- 75 mg of vitamin C
- 1000 mg of calcium

To reach those nutritional goals, each day you should eat approximately:

- 6 ounces of grains and grain foods like breads and cereals, with at least half being whole grain
- 2½ cups of different kinds of veggies
- 2 cups of fruit
- 3 cups of milk or other calcium-rich beverages
- 5½ ounces of protein foods

They will be spread out in your meals like so:

	Maintain Meal Plan	Include These Types of Food
Breakfast	450 calories	Grain, fruit, dairy, and/or protein
Lunch & Dinner	525 calories	Vegetables, protein, grain, fruit, and/or dairy
Snack	2 x 250 calories	Fruit, vegetables, grain, and/or protein

Maintain Breakfasts

Breakfast #1

1 cup Life cereal topped with ½ cup raspberries, 2 Tbsp sliced almonds, and 1 cup fat-free milk

1 5.2–6 oz carton (80–100 calories) Greek yogurt

428 calories

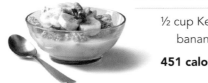

Breakfast #2

½ cup Kellogg's Frosted Mini Wheats topped with 1 medium banana, 1½ Tbsp walnuts, and 1 cup fat-free milk

451 calories

Breakfast #3

1 packet (1.75 oz) Nature's Path Organic Instant Maple Nut Hot Oatmeal topped with 2 Tbsp pecans and 2 Tbsp chopped dried fruit

1 cup fat-free milk

428 calories

Breakfast #4

Jamba Juice Steel-Cut Oatmeal with blueberries and strawberries

16 oz Jamba Juice Strawberries Wild Smoothie

455 calories

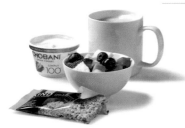

Breakfast #5

KIND Healthy Grains bar, any flavor

1 5.2–6 oz carton (80–100 calories) Greek yogurt

1 cup fruit salad

16 oz latte made with 1 cup each hot fat-free milk and coffee

460 calories

Breakfast #6

1 package belVita Soft Baked Cinnamon Breakfast Biscuits

2 Mini Babybel Light cheeses

1 medium apple

425 calories

Breakfast #7

Tim Horton Egg Cheese Grilled Breakfast Wrap

16 oz Tim Horton Iced Latte

440 calories

Breakfast #8

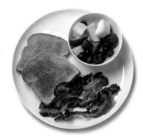

3 slices bacon

2 slices whole wheat toast

1 cup fruit salad

451 calories

Breakfast #9

2 slices Freihofer Hearty 100% Whole Wheat with Honey topped with 2 Tbsp
almond butter and 4 peach slices (½ cup)

442 calories

Breakfast #10

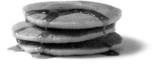

Burger King Pancakes with syrup, no butter or sausage

420 calories

Breakfast #11

Panera Orange Mini Scone

Medium (16 oz) Panera Low-Fat Mango Smoothie

450 calories

Breakfast #12

Dunkin' Donuts Jelly Donut

Dunkin' Donuts Large Latte Lite

410 calories

Breakfast #13

Good Food Made Simple Turkey Sausage Breakfast Burrito

1 6-oz carton Yoplait Light yogurt, any flavor

½ cup blueberries

432 calories

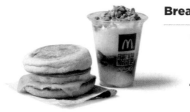

Breakfast #14

McDonald's Egg McMuffin

McDonald's Fruit 'n Yogurt Parfait

450 calories

Breakfast #15

Panera Avocado, Egg White & Spinach Breakfast Power Sandwich

Small Panera coffee with fat-free milk

435 calories

Breakfast #16

2-egg omelet with 2 Tbsp Sargento Shredded Reduced Fat 4 Cheese
Mexican cheese and ½ cup broccoli, cooked in a nonstick pan

2 slices Freihofer Hearty 100% Whole Wheat Bread

410 calories

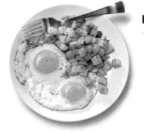

Breakfast #17

1 cup home fries

2 eggs, any way you like them (sunny-side up, sunny-side
down, scrambled, fried, or poached)

432 calories

Breakfast #18

¾ cup 1% cottage cheese in ½ small cantaloupe

1 muffin prepared from Krusteaz Honey Cornbread Muffin Mix, with 1 tsp butter

410 calories

Breakfast #19

Juice made with:

   1 cup kale, chopped

   1 medium apple, peeled, cored, and chopped

   1 medium carrot, peeled and chopped

   1 mandarin orange, peeled

   1 Tbsp almond or peanut butter

   1-inch piece fresh ginger, peeled and chopped

Thomas' 100% Whole Wheat Bagel Thins bagel with 1 Tbsp light cream cheese

429 calories

Breakfast #20

16 oz Jamba Juice Amazing Greens Smoothie

420 calories

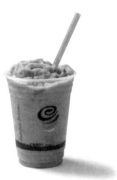

Maintain Lunches

Lunch #1

Ready Pac Bistro Bowl Chicken Caesar Salad
  (note that this is not the Organic or Lite Salad)

Rudi's Organic Whole Grain Wheat English Muffins

1 clementine orange

1 mini cupcake (1 oz)

495 calories

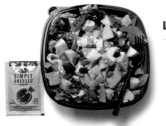

Lunch #2

Wendy's Apple Pecan Chicken Salad with 1 packet
  Pomegranate Vinaigrette

530 calories

Lunch #3

Panera half-size Chicken Cobb Salad with Avocado with 1½ Tbsp (½ portion)
  Panera Reduced Fat Balsamic Vinaigrette

1 Panera Petite Chocolate Chipper

520 calories

Lunch #4

Chef's salad made with 1 oz slice each turkey, ham, and reduced-fat Swiss
  cheese, 1 hard-boiled egg, 2 cups lettuce or mixed greens, 4 tomato
  wedges, and 2 Tbsp reduced-fat ranch dressing

Thomas' High Fiber English Muffin

3 Keebler Fudge Shoppe Cheesecake Middles Original Graham cookies

518 calories

Lunch #5

Arby's Roast Beef Classic Sandwich

Arby's Chopped Side Salad with 1 packet Light Italian dressing

1 Arby's Jalapeño Bite (5 come per order; share or save the rest)

506 calories

Lunch #6

6-inch whole wheat pita filled with ½ cup hummus, 2 Tbsp chopped tomato, ¼ cup lettuce, and ½ cup sliced cucumbers drizzled with vinegar and a pinch of noncaloric sweetener if desired

Skinny Cow Vanilla Ice Cream Sandwich

537 calories

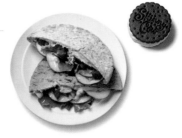

Lunch #7

Wrap made with La Tortilla Factory Traditional Sonoma Organic Wrap, 2 1-oz slices Monterey Jack cheese, 2 Tbsp chopped tomato, ¼ cup lettuce, and 2 Tbsp Wholly Guacamole Classic

1 cup watermelon cubes

518 calories

Lunch #8

½ Panera Classic Grilled Cheese

½ Panera Greek Salad with 1½ Tbsp (½ portion) Panera Reduced Fat Balsamic Vinaigrette

530 calories

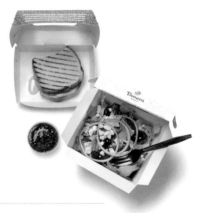

Lunch #9

Sonic All Beef Regular Hot Dog with mustard

Sonic Vanilla Dish (ice cream)

560 calories

Lunch #10

3 Chick-fil-A Chick-n-Strips

1 packet Chick-fil-A Barbeque Sauce

Chick-fil-A Side Salad with 1 packet Light Italian Dressing

Chick-fil-A Small Fruit Cup

555 calories

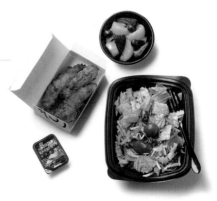

Lunch #11

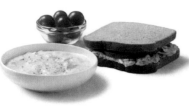

1 cup (½ can) Progresso Traditional New England Clam Chowder

Tuna salad (⅓ cup tuna in water with 1½ Tbsp light mayo and 2 Tbsp chopped celery) on 2 slices Pepperidge Farm Whole Grain Honey Oat Bread with lettuce and tomato

½ cup cherry tomatoes

526 calories

Lunch #12

2 cups (1 can) Amy's Organic Split Pea Soup

11 (1 oz; ⅑ bag) New York Style Sea Salt Pita Chips

1 cup mixed greens with 2 Tbsp light Caesar dressing

1 cup pineapple chunks

492 calories

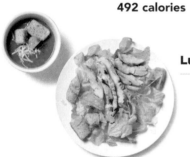

Lunch #13

Applebee's lunch menu Tomato Basil Soup

Applebee's lunch menu Grilled Chicken Caesar Salad

510 calories

Lunch #14

1 bowl TGI Friday's French Onion Soup

⅓ order TGI Friday's Spinach Florentine Flatbread

TGI Friday's Side Salad with 2 Tbsp (½ serving) Caesar Vinaigrette

537 calories

Lunch #15

1 cup (½ can) Campbell's Chunky Savory Vegetable Soup

Banquet Turkey Meal

1 medium (2½-inch) whole wheat roll

1 cup fruit salad

516 calories

Lunch #16

1 cup (⅙ recipe) homemade chili made with 1 pound 90% lean ground beef, 1 15–16 oz can chili beans, 1 Tbsp chili powder, 1 15–16 oz can tomatoes with green chiles, and 1 cup diced tomatoes topped with 2 Tbsp plain 0% Greek yogurt and 2 Tbsp Kraft Shredded Reduced Fat Mild Cheddar

½ cup cooked white rice

2 cups lettuce or mixed greens, sprinkled with vinegar and 4 sprays of olive oil

1 medium orange

519 calories

Lunch #17

CedarLane Eggplant Parmesan

1 cup fresh greens of your choice (kale, spinach, chard, bok choy, etc.) and 1 tsp chopped garlic (optional), sautéed with ½ tsp olive oil

2 thin slices Italian bread

½ cup raspberries

515 calories

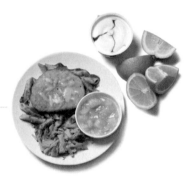

Lunch #18

Healthy Choice Chicken Parmigiana

1 4-oz cup Healthy Choice Frozen Yogurt, any flavor

1 medium orange

509 calories

Lunch #19

½ California Pizza Kitchen Wild Mushroom Pizza

515 calories

Lunch #20

⅓ Newman's Own Uncured Pepperoni Thin & Crispy Pizza

1 cup steamed broccoli

½ cup (1 container) Kozy Shack Simply Well Rice Pudding topped with 2 Tbsp sliced almonds

531 calories

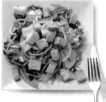

Maintain Dinners

Dinner #1

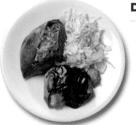

¼ order Chili's Classic Nachos

Chili's Lighter Choice Margarita Grilled Chicken, no sides

Chili's House Salad, sprinkled with vinegar

548 calories

Dinner #2

Bertolli Rustico Bakes Chicken Parmigiana & Penne meal

2 cups baby lettuce, sprinkled with vinegar and 4 sprays of olive oil

Nestlé Outshine Strawberry Fruit Bar

525 calories

Dinner #3

½ order PF Chang's Almond and Cashew Chicken

Small PF Chang's Spicy Green Beans

530 calories

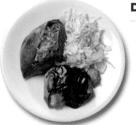

Dinner #4

4 oz roasted chicken thigh, no skin, with 1 Tbsp barbecue sauce

1 medium roasted sweet potato

½ cup no-mayo coleslaw

522 calories

Dinner #5

4 oz grilled chicken breast

1 small baked potato with 1 Tbsp light sour cream

1 cup steamed carrots

½ cup Ciao Bella Alphonso Mango Sorbetto

522 calories

Dinner #6

½ order Applebee's Artisan Grilled Chicken Ciabatta

Applebee's Seasonal Vegetables side dish

530 calories

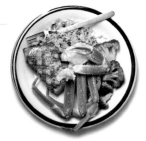

Dinner #7

6 oz tilapia fillet cooked in ½ cup Patak's Mild Curry Simmer Sauce

½ cup cooked quinoa

1 cup steamed cauliflower

½ cup mango slices

518 calories

Dinner #8

Red Lobster Create Your Own Combination portion
    Wood-Grilled Fresh Salmon

Red Lobster Create Your Own Combination portion
    Steamed Snow Crab Legs

Red Lobster Broccoli

Red Lobster Wild Rice Pilaf

530 calories

Dinner #9

½ order Legal Sea Foods Lobster Ravioli "Fra Diavolo"

532 calories

Dinner #10

1 Sloppy Joe (⅛ recipe) made with 1 pound 90% lean ground beef,
    1 package McCormick Sloppy Joes Seasoning Mix, 1 can (6 oz) tomato
    paste, and 1¼ cups water and served on a whole wheat hamburger bun

3 oz (⅐ package) Ore-Ida Extra Crispy Fast Food Fries with 1 Tbsp ketchup

10 medium baby carrots with 2 Tbsp Wholly Guacamole Classic

½ cup strawberries

528 calories

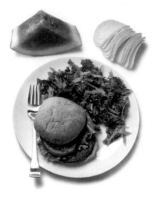

Dinner #11

1 Boca All American Flame Grilled Veggie Burger on a whole wheat burger bun with lettuce and tomato

1½ cups Cut'N Clean SuperKALE Salad Slaw tossed with vinegar and 1 tsp olive oil

16 (about ⅓ can) Pringles Original Fat-Free Potato Crisps

1 slice watermelon

525 calories

Dinner #12

½ cup (¼ package) firm tofu and 1½ cups frozen Asian vegetables stir-fried in 1 tsp oil, with 1 Tbsp teriyaki sauce

½ cup cooked brown rice

4 oz (less than ½ of a 10-oz package) edamame

½ cup fat-free vanilla frozen yogurt

524 calories

Dinner #13

Benihana Hibachi Steak

½ order Benihana Brown Rice

Benihana Salad with dressing

495 calories

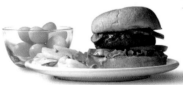

Dinner #14

4 oz 95% lean ground beef patty on a whole wheat burger bun, topped with 1 Tbsp ketchup, ½ cup mushrooms sautéed in ½ tsp olive oil, lettuce, tomato, and pickles

½ cup deli German potato salad

½ cup grapes

525 calories

Dinner #15

On the Border Green Chile Carnitas Taco (ask for half the rice)

On the Border Grilled Vegetables

½ order On the Border Black Beans

520 calories

Dinner #16

4 oz grilled pork tenderloin

1 cup prepared (from ¼ box) Idahoan Au Gratin
Homestyle Casserole

¾ cup steamed carrots

Klondike No Sugar Added Krunch bar

524 calories

Dinner #17

Small order Bonefish Grill Chilean Sea Bass

½ order Bonefish Grill Herbed Couscous

Bonefish Grill Steamed Asparagus

537 calories

Dinner #18

1 cup cooked linguine topped with ½ cup (⅓ can) Cento
White Clam Sauce

¾ cup steamed broccoli

1 cup (½ can) Progresso Vegetable Classics Minestrone

523 calories

Dinner #19

Banquet Fettuccine Alfredo

1 medium tomato, sliced, with 2 thin slices (1 oz) fresh mozzarella cheese and
fresh basil

1 cup steamed broccoli

2 Trader Joe's Soft Bite Mini Almond Biscotti

536 calories

Dinner #20

½ order Maggiano's Mushroom Ravioli al Forno

1 Maggiano's Chocolate Zuccotto Bite

515 calories

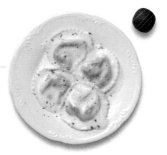

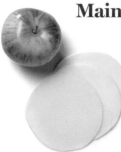

Maintain Snacks

Snack #1

1 medium apple

3 slices (57 g) Sargento Thin Sliced Reduced Fat Provolone

245 calories

Snack #2

1 small banana, sliced into rounds, topped with ½ tsp brown sugar and
½ tsp butter, and microwaved until soft, about 30 seconds

½ cup fat-free vanilla frozen yogurt

230 calories

Snack #3

20 Trader Joe's Peanut Butter Filled Pretzels

254 calories

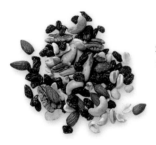

Snack #4

¼ cup roasted mixed nuts with 2 Tbsp raisins

224 calories

Snack #5

Clif Dark Chocolate Peanut Butter bar

½ cup fat-free milk

240 calories

Snack #6

Nature Valley Sweet & Salty Nut Dark Chocolate,
  Peanut & Almond Granola Bar

1 small banana

250 calories

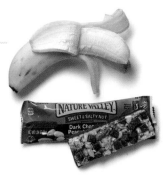

Snack #7

1 oz bag Pirate's Booty Smart Puffs Real Wisconsin Cheddar

1 medium apple

235 calories

Snack #8

61 (1 oz; about ⅕ container) EatSmart Snacks Sea Salt
  Garden Veggie Sticks

¼ cup (about ¼ of an 8-oz carton) Tribe Sweet
  Roasted Red Pepper Hummus

230 calories

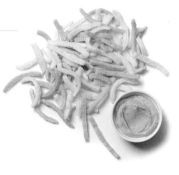

Snack #9

½ cup (¼ recipe) salsa made with 1 chopped medium tomato, 1 chopped
  avocado, 2 Tbsp minced onion, juice of ½ lime, salt to taste, and chopped
  jalapeño and cilantro if desired

10 (1 oz) Food Should Taste Good Multi-Grain Tortilla Chips

230 calories

Snack #10

11 (1 oz; ⅟₇ bag) Snack Factory Pretzel Crisps Original

2 Mini Babybel Light cheeses

250 calories

Snack #11

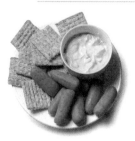

¼ cup (⅛ recipe) onion dip made with 1 packet Lipton Recipe Secrets Onion Dip Mix and 2 cups 0% plain fat Greek yogurt

8 baby carrots

8 Reduced Fat Triscuit crackers

228 calories

Snack #12

½ order California Pizza Kitchen White Corn Guacamole & Chips

205 calories

Snack #13

½ order Applebee's Grilled Chicken Wonton Tacos

230 calories

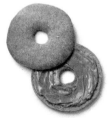

Snack #14

Thomas' 100% Whole Wheat Bagel Thins bagel with 1½ Tbsp peanut butter

251 calories

Snack #15

1 container Spice Hunter Reduced Sodium Split Pea Vegetarian Soup Cup

1 slice Wasa Multi-Grain Crispbread

250 calories

Snack #16

½ Starbucks Cheese & Fruit Bistro Box

240 calories

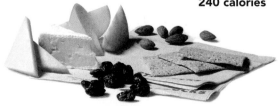

Snack #17

16 oz Red Mango Strawberry-Banana Fruit & Yogurt Smoothie

240 calories

Snack #18

1 3.9-oz carton Breakstone's Strawberry Cottage Doubles

1 5.2–6 oz carton (80–100 calories) yogurt

1 slice Wasa Fiber Crispbread

240 calories

Snack #19

¼ cup Sabra Cucumber Dill Greek Yogurt Dip

40 (1 oz, ¼ bag) Food Should Taste Good Chive Pita Puffs

210 calories

Snack #20

1 piece (2 oz) Panera Cinnamon Crumb Coffee Cake

220 calories

Snack #21

9 Hershey's Special Dark Kisses

½ cup fat-free milk

230 calories

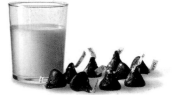

Snack #22

4 Ghirardelli Milk & Caramel squares

240 calories

Part Three

THE FOODS

Part Three is your guide to making the best choices for health and weight loss, no matter what you're craving or where you're eating. For more than 75 everyday foods from eggs to chicken noodle soup to mac 'n' cheese, we list recipes, brand-name products, and restaurant dishes you should stop eating. Then you'll see similar options to start eating instead. We marked the phase in which they can fit and photographed the package as you'll see it in the grocery store or the dish as it's served in the restaurant. Because the photos were intended to help you quickly recognize the food when you buy or order it, they do not necessarily show the portion you should eat. (You'll only eat one Oscar Meyer hot dog, for instance, but we show the whole package of eight. You'll eat two slices of Pizza Hut pizza, but we show the whole pie.)

In some cases, there isn't a huge calorie difference between the Stop Eating and Start Eating choices. That's because we also considered the amount and type of fat, sugar, sodium, and other nutrients in the foods and have highlighted them when they are significant. For the same reason, you may also sometimes see that a Kickstart choice has more calories than a Steady Loss or Maintain option.

You'll also see that sometimes the Stop Eating and Start Eating choices have different portions. It might not seem fair to compare a whole package of Sabra Classic Hummus with Pretzels, for instance, to a mere 2 tablespoons of Athenos Roasted Red Pepper Hummus. But too many people *will* mindlessly polish off an entire package, which is exactly what you need to stop doing.

By no means are these comprehensive lists. Remember that just because a brand or restaurant you like has a food in the Stop Eating list doesn't mean it's completely unhealthy; similarly, just because a brand or restaurant has a food in the Start Eating list doesn't mean everything it offers is healthy. The key is to look at each individual product or dish and the portions for each.

Chapter 8
BREAKFAST FOODS

Good morning! I am a breakfast believer. As a working mom, I need to start every day with my feet on the ground and my body rested and energized. That doesn't happen if I don't eat breakfast. You'll see from the choices in this chapter that Stop & Drop breakfasts don't take much time to prepare. With a selection of convenience foods, restaurant offerings, and meals to make at home, you're bound to find foods that fit your routine and taste buds.

My biggest personal rule is to stop eating carb-only breakfasts. They might give me a quick rush, but they're missing the protein I need for energy in the morning. I also hit a wall midmorning if my breakfast foods are highly sweetened. The sugar adds calories, doesn't help fill me up, and sends my blood sugar crashing after just a couple of hours. That doesn't mean you can never have a doughnut again; in fact, while I wouldn't suggest making these your go-to breakfasts, you'll see I offer some smarter choices for doughnuts as well as muffins, scones, and other breakfast pastries—even Pop-Tarts!

If you do opt for a high-carb food for breakfast, though, take a look at the meals in Chapters 5, 6, and 7 for ideas on how to balance them with other foods that supply protein and/or healthy fats, such as eggs, dairy, and nut butters. You can also add some lean meats like turkey, chicken sausage, or Canadian bacon; I don't recommend many traditional breakfast meats, such as regular bacon, sausage, or corned beef hash, which all tend to be high in saturated fats and, of course, calories. (And beware of foods with added protein, such as high-protein cereals or bars. All too often, the added protein also adds calories.) Even on the Kickstart phase, you can get a good mix. In Kickstart Breakfast #3, for instance, you'll top oatmeal with pecans for healthy fats and enjoy yogurt with your meal for protein. Keep in mind that it's most important to balance your nutrition over the course of the day. So if you have a high-carb breakfast, opt for a lower-carb lunch and dinner that day.

I also make sure I fit in calcium. Experts recommend that we get at least 1000 mg of calcium in our diet every day—that's the equivalent of three servings of milk or other calcium-containing drinks and foods. Having milk or yogurt at breakfast gets me started toward my goal. It's best to opt for milks and yogurts that don't have extra calories from fat and sugars.

Remember to watch your portions, as breakfast foods, especially breads and pastries, are often oversized. The average bagel shop bagel is the equivalent of four slices of bread, and a large muffin can match the calories in a piece of cake. And have you considered how much cream cheese is spread onto a bagel?! I've mapped out portions for you, but be sure to look at the "Portion Guide" on page 9 to help you make smart choices when you're eating away from home.

Also, when you eat at a restaurant for breakfast, avoid extras like potatoes, butter, jam, and other items that might be available with your dish. Throughout this chapter, I let you know which sides can be part of your meal.

STOP EATING	START EATING
• Carb-only breakfasts that don't fill you up and mess up your morning energy levels	• Protein-packed breakfast foods that are satisfying and keep you going for longer
• Nutrient-poor breakfast foods and drinks	• Foods and drinks that deliver important vitamins and minerals, including calcium
• Excess calories from high-fat spreads like butter	• Measured portions of peanut butter, almond butter, and other tummy-trimming MUFA-rich spreads
• Oversized bagels and muffins with too many calories for one meal	• Smaller bagels, mini muffins, and other portion-controlled breakfast breads
• Indulgent restaurant breakfast plates with generous portions of eggs, bread, potatoes, and meats	• A la carte ordering off the restaurant menu

Breakfast Foods
CEREALS

❌ STOP EATING	✅ START EATING

🛒 Packaged

❌ ½ cup Grape-Nuts
(210 calories)

❌ 1¼ cups Cheerios
Protein Oats & Honey
(210 calories, 17 g sugars)

❌ 1 cup Barbara's Morning
Oat Crunch Original
(210 calories, 12 g sugars)

✔ ¾ cup Total Whole
Grain **KICK START**

100 calories

✔ 1¼ cups Kix **KICK START**

110 calories
3 g fiber

Choose Your Milk

What you eat your cereal with can make a big difference. See how many calories per cup you get with different types of milks and milk alternatives.

Whole milk	149	Fat-free milk	83
2% milk	122	Silk Original Almond Milk	60
Skim Plus milk	110	Coconut Dream Unsweetened Coconut Milk	60
Low-fat (1% fat) milk	102	Silk Light Original Soymilk	60

✅ START EATING

🛒 *Packaged*

✔ ¾ cup Kellogg's
All-Bran Original

KICK START

120 calories
15 g fiber

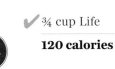

✔ ¾ cup Life

120 calories

KICK START

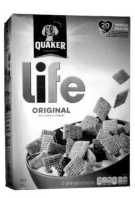

Other Good Choices

✔ ½ cup Fiber One Original
(60 calories, 14 g fiber)

✔ ¾ cup Kellogg's All-Bran
Complete Wheat Flakes
(90 calories)

✔ 1 cup Cascadian Farm
Honey Nut O's
(110 calories)

✔ ¾ cup Nature's Path Flax
Plus Flakes **(110 calories,
5 g fiber)**

✔ ¾ cup Wheat Chex
(160 calories)

✔ ¾ cup Kashi GOLEAN
Crunch!

STEADY LOSS

190 calories
9 g protein

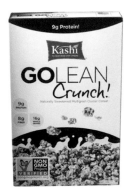

✔ ½ cup Kellogg's Frosted
Mini Wheats

STEADY LOSS

190 calories
6 g fiber

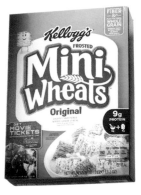

Breakfast Foods
GRANOLA AND GRANOLA BARS

❌ STOP EATING	✅ START EATING

🛒 *Packaged*

STOP EATING

❌ ⅔ cup Cascadian Farm Fruit and Nut Granola (230 calories, 17 g sugars)

❌ ⅓ cup Go Raw Super Simple Granola (230 calories)

❌ 1 pouch Larabar Cinnamon Nut Renola (200 calories, 14 g fat)

START EATING

✅ Quaker Chewy Chocolate Chip Granola Bar **KICK START**

100 calories

✅ ¼ cup Nature's Path Fruit & Nut Granola **KICK START**

140 calories
5 g fat

✅ ¼ cup Bear Naked Fruit and Nutty Goodie Bag Granola **KICK START**

140 calories

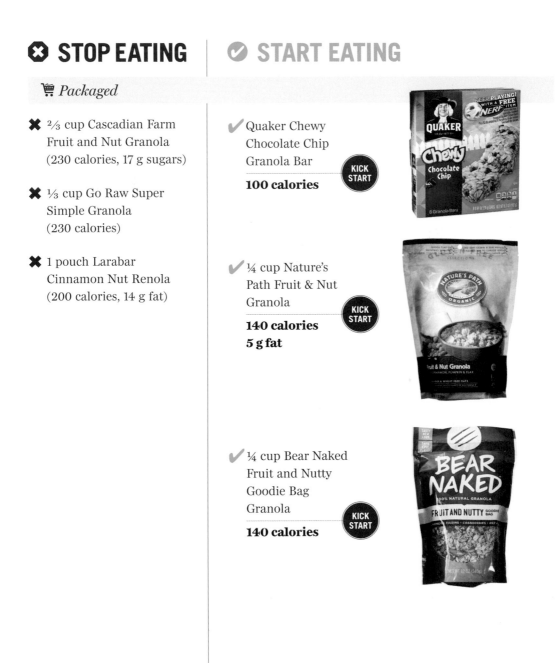

✅ START EATING

🛒 *Packaged*

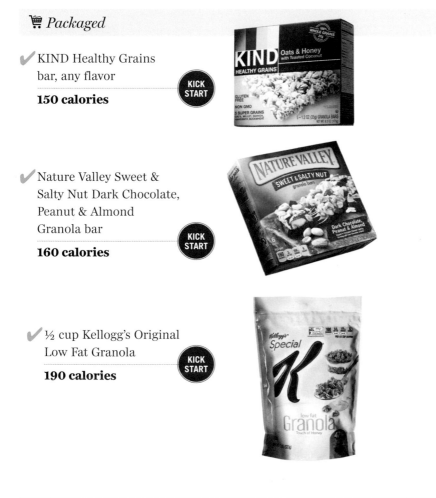

✔ KIND Healthy Grains
bar, any flavor

150 calories

(KICK START)

✔ Nature Valley Sweet &
Salty Nut Dark Chocolate,
Peanut & Almond
Granola bar

160 calories

(KICK START)

✔ ½ cup Kellogg's Original
Low Fat Granola

190 calories

(KICK START)

Other Good Choices

✓ Nature Valley Oats 'n Honey Crunchy Granola Bar (1 bar, ½ pouch) **(90 calories, 3 g fat)**

✓ Kellogg's Special K Protein Almond Honey Oat Granola Bar **(110 calories)**

✓ Kashi Honey Almond Flax Chewy Granola Bar **(140 calories, 5 g fat)**

✓ Fiber One Chewy Protein Bar **(140 calories, 6 g fat)**

Breakfast Foods
OATMEAL AND GRITS

❌ STOP EATING	✓ START EATING

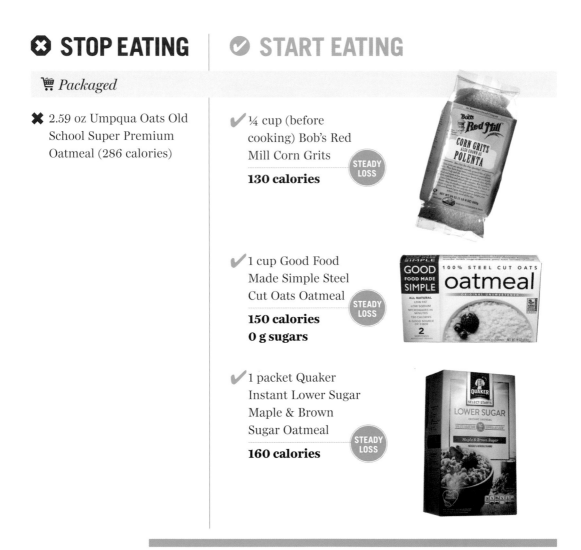

🛒 *Packaged*

STOP EATING:

✖ 2.59 oz Umpqua Oats Old School Super Premium Oatmeal (286 calories)

START EATING:

✓ ¼ cup (before cooking) Bob's Red Mill Corn Grits

STEADY LOSS

130 calories

✓ 1 cup Good Food Made Simple Steel Cut Oats Oatmeal

STEADY LOSS

150 calories
0 g sugars

✓ 1 packet Quaker Instant Lower Sugar Maple & Brown Sugar Oatmeal

STEADY LOSS

160 calories

Other Good Choices

✓ 1 packet plain Quaker Instant Original Oatmeal (**100 calories**)

✓ 1 packet Quaker Butter Flavor Instant Grits (**100 calories**)

✓ ½ cup McCann's Quick Cooking Irish Oatmeal (**150 calories**)

✓ 1 packet Kashi Heart to Heart Golden Maple Instant Oatmeal (**150 calories, 5 g fiber**)

✓ 1.75 oz Nature's Path Organic Instant Maple Nut Hot Oatmeal (**210 calories**)

✖ STOP EATING | ✔ START EATING

✗ *Restaurant*

✖ Caribou Coffee Maple
Brown Sugar Crunch
Oatmeal (320 calories,
16 g sugars)

✖ McDonald's Fruit
& Maple Oatmeal
(290 calories)

✔ Burger King Original Maple Flavored
Quaker Oatmeal

170 calories

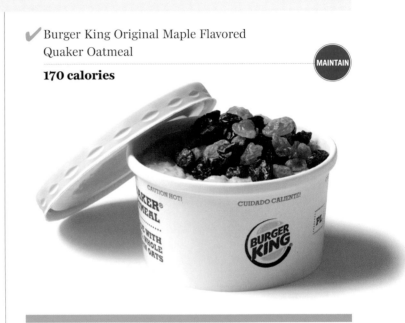

MAINTAIN

Other Good Choices

✓ Starbucks Classic Whole-Grain Oatmeal **(160 calories)**

✓ Small Au Bon Pain Apple Cinnamon Oatmeal **(190 calories)**

✓ Jamba Juice Steel-Cut Oatmeal with blueberries, strawberries
(195 calories)

Choose Your Toppings

When it comes to oatmeal and grits, simpler is better. See how many calories per tablespoon your
favorite oatmeal toppings have.

Butter	102	Chopped pecans	47	Shredded coconut	29
Maple syrup	52	Brown sugar	34	Seedless raisins	27
Chopped walnuts	48	Sliced almonds	33	Chopped apple	4

BREAKFAST BREADS

❌ STOP EATING	✅ START EATING

🛒 *Packaged*

❌ Bruegger's Whole Wheat Bagel (270 calories)

❌ Thomas' Double Protein English Muffin (150 calories, 1 g fiber)

❌ 1 slice Pepperidge Farm Farmhouse Honey Wheat Bread (120 calories)

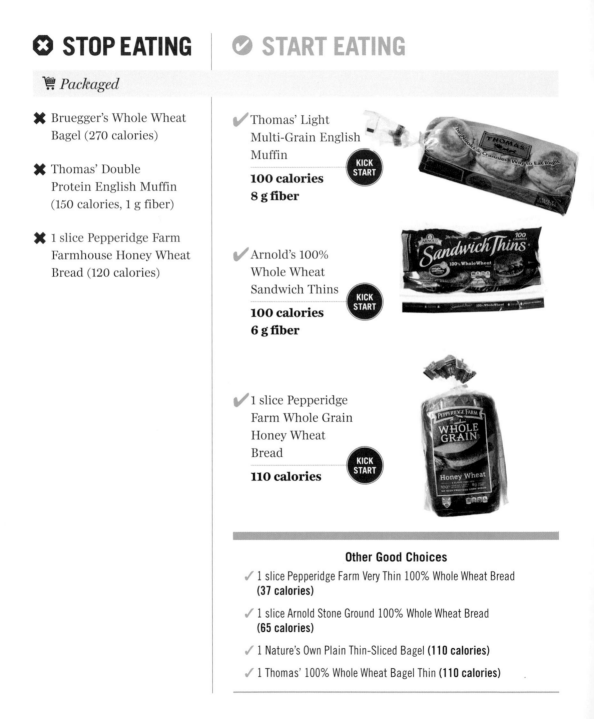

✔ Thomas' Light Multi-Grain English Muffin

100 calories
8 g fiber

KICK START

✔ Arnold's 100% Whole Wheat Sandwich Thins

100 calories
6 g fiber

KICK START

✔ 1 slice Pepperidge Farm Whole Grain Honey Wheat Bread

110 calories

KICK START

Other Good Choices

✓ 1 slice Pepperidge Farm Very Thin 100% Whole Wheat Bread **(37 calories)**

✓ 1 slice Arnold Stone Ground 100% Whole Wheat Bread **(65 calories)**

✓ 1 Nature's Own Plain Thin-Sliced Bagel **(110 calories)**

✓ 1 Thomas' 100% Whole Wheat Bagel Thin **(110 calories)**

✖ STOP EATING | ✔ START EATING

✗ Restaurant

✖ Dunkin' Donuts Multigrain Bagel (350 calories)

✖ Einstein Bros. Bagels Honey Whole Wheat Bagel (260 calories)

✔ Einstein Bros. Bagels Honey Whole Wheat Bagel (ask for a "thin" bagel)

160 calories

KICK START

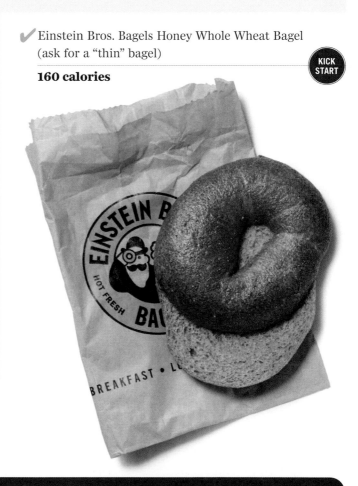

Choose Your Spreads

Think cream cheese is the worst? Think again! See how many calories are in your favorite spreads, per teaspoon.

Butter...34	Peanut butter.............................31	Cream cheese.............................17
Smart Balance Original buttery spread............................33	I Can't Believe It's Not Butter.....30	All-fruit jam................................13
	Jam...19	Low-fat cream cheese................10

Breakfast Foods
PASTRIES

❌ **STOP EATING**	✅ **START EATING**

🛒 *Packaged*

❌ 1 muffin made from Krusteaz Banana Nut Muffin Mix (250 calories)

❌ 1 Kellogg's Brown Sugar Cinnamon Pop-Tart (210 calories)

✅ 1 muffin made from Fiber One Blueberry Muffin Mix

STEADY LOSS

160 calories
5 g fiber

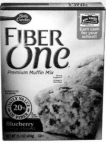

✅ 1 Kellogg's Low Fat Frosted Brown Sugar Cinnamon with Whole Grain and Fiber Pop-Tart

STEADY LOSS

180 calories

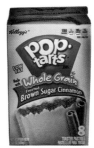

Other Good Choices

✓ 2 Kellogg's Special K Brown Sugar Cinnamon Pastry Crisps **(100 calories)**

✓ 1 muffin made from Krusteaz Fat Free Banana Muffin Mix **(140 calories, 0 g fat)**

✓ 1 muffin made from Jiffy Corn Muffin mix **(170 calories)**

✘ STOP EATING | ✔ START EATING

✘ Panera Orange Scone (540 calories, 38 g sugars)

✘ Au Bon Pain Blueberry Muffin (490 calories, 19 g fat)

✔ Dunkin' Donuts Jelly Donut

270 calories

MAINTAIN

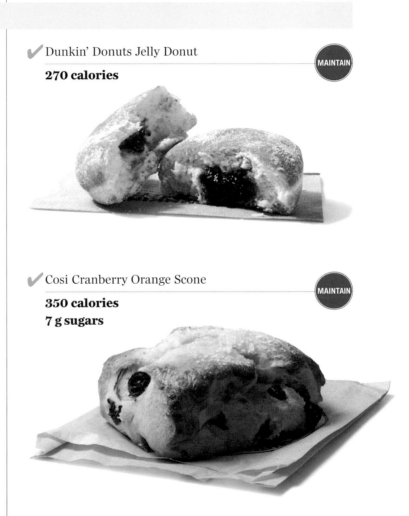

✔ Cosi Cranberry Orange Scone

350 calories

7 g sugars

MAINTAIN

Other Good Choices

✓ Panera Orange Mini Scone **(180 calories, 13 g sugars)**

✓ Dunkin' Donuts Apple 'n' Spice Donut **(260 calories, 9 g sugars)**

✓ Au Bon Pain Low Fat Berry Muffin **(290 calories, 3 g fat)**

Breakfast Foods
PANCAKES AND WAFFLES

❌ STOP EATING | ✅ START EATING

🛒 Packaged

❌ 2 pancakes made from Arrowhead Mills Buckwheat Pancake and Waffle Mix (320 calories, 12 g fat)

❌ 3 Kellogg's Eggo Buttermilk Pancakes (280 calories, 12 g sugars)

❌ 3 pancakes made from Bisquick Complete Simply Buttermilk with Whole Grain Pancake and Waffle Mix (210 calories)

✅ 2 pancakes made from Aunt Jemima Complete Pancake and Waffle Mix

160 calories

STEADY LOSS

✅ 2 Van's 8 Whole Grains Pancakes

160 calories
5 g fiber

STEADY LOSS

✅ 2 Kellogg's Eggo Nutri-Grain Whole Wheat Waffles

170 calories
3 g sugars

STEADY LOSS

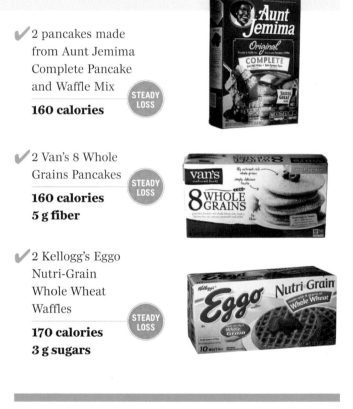

Other Good Choices

✓ 2 Van's 8 Whole Grains Waffles (**150 calories, 2 g sugars**)

✓ 2 Kashi 7 Grain Waffles (**150 calories, 3 g sugars**)

✓ 3 pancakes made from Krusteaz Buttermilk Complete Pancake Mix (**180 calories, 6 g sugars**)

❌ STOP EATING | ✓ START EATING

✗ *Restaurant*

❌ 1 IHOP Belgian Waffle
(500 calories, 14 g
sugars)

✓ 1 Perkins Belgian
Waffle

MAINTAIN

**350 calories
2 g sugars**

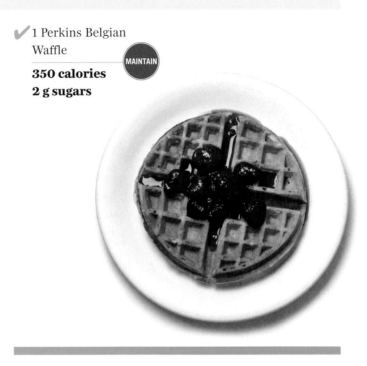

Other Good Choices

✓ Bob Evans Belgian Waffle **(351 calories, 1 g sugars)**

✓ Burger King Pancakes with syrup, no butter or sausage
(420 calories)

Choose Your Toppings

See how many calories are in your favorite toppings, per tablespoon.

Nutella 100	Chocolate syrup........................... 54	Almond syrup 45
Agave syrup................................. 64	Maple-flavored syrup 53	Sugar-free almond syrup.............. 0
Honey 64	Maple syrup................................ 52	

Breakfast Foods
BREAKFAST SANDWICHES AND WRAPS

❌ STOP EATING	✅ START EATING

🛒 *Packaged*

✖ Jimmy Dean Delights
Sausage, Egg & Cheese
Biscuit Sandwich
(410 calories, 29 g fat)

✔ Jimmy Dean
Delights Bacon,
Egg & Cheese
Honey Wheat
Flatbread — **KICK START**

230 calories
12 g fat

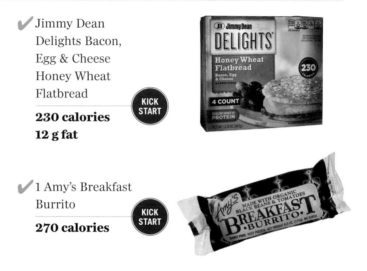

✔ 1 Amy's Breakfast
Burrito — **KICK START**

270 calories

Other Good Choices

✓ Weight Watchers Smart Ones Smart Beginnings Canadian Style
Turkey Bacon English Muffin Sandwich **(210 calories, 6 g fat)**

✓ Atkins Canadian Bacon with Egg and Cheese English Muffin
Sandwich **(230 calories, 14 g fat)**

✓ Amy's Southwestern Burrito **(290 calories)**

✓ Good Food Made Simple Turkey Sausage Breakfast Burrito
(300 calories)

✓ Good Food Made Simple Chicken Apple Sausage Egg White
Breakfast Burrito **(310 calories)**

✖ STOP EATING | ✔ START EATING

✗ *Restaurant*

✖ Arby's Sausage, Egg & Cheese Biscuit (620 calories, 43 g fat)

✖ Au Bon Pain Eggs on a Bagel with Bacon and Cheese (560 calories, 22 g fat)

✔ McDonald's Egg McMuffin

300 calories

STEADY LOSS

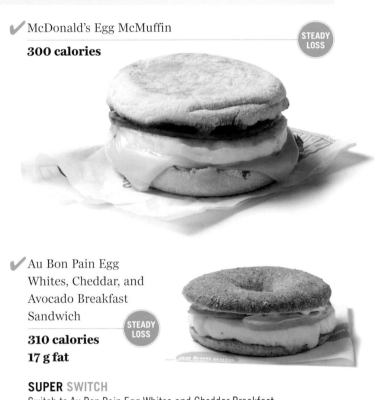

✔ Au Bon Pain Egg Whites, Cheddar, and Avocado Breakfast Sandwich

STEADY LOSS

310 calories
17 g fat

SUPER SWITCH
Switch to Au Bon Pain Egg Whites and Cheddar Breakfast Sandwich and drop another 80 calories and 8 g fat!

Other Good Choices

✓ Starbucks Reduced Fat Turkey Bacon Breakfast Sandwich **(230 calories, 6 g fat)**

✓ Tim Horton Egg Cheese Grilled Breakfast Wrap **(230 calories, 12 g fat)**

✓ Starbucks Spinach & Feta Breakfast Wrap **(290 calories)**

✓ Taco Bell Cheesy Steak and Egg Fresco Style Burrito **(320 calories)**

✓ Panera Avocado, Egg White & Spinach Breakfast Power Sandwich **(440 calories)**

Breakfast Foods
EGGS

⊗ **STOP EATING**	⊘ **START EATING**

🏠 *Homemade*

✖ 3 scrambled eggs with 1 slice cheddar cheese (387 calories, 29.5 g fat)

✔ 2 scrambled eggs with 1 Tbsp grated cheddar cheese

STEADY LOSS

210 calories
16 g fat

🛒 *Packaged*

✖ Jimmy Dean Meat Lovers Breakfast Bowl (460 calories, 33 g fat)

✖ Atkins Farmhouse-Style Sausage Scramble (370 calories, 29 g fat)

✖ Marie Callender's frozen Breakfast Anytime! Egg, Cheese & Ham Bake (330 calories, 19 g fat)

✔ CedarLane Spinach & Roasted Tomato Egg White Frittata

STEADY LOSS

160 calories
6 g fat

✔ Jimmy Dean Three Cheese Omelet

MAINTAIN

290 calories
23 g fat

Other Good Choices

✓ Weight Watchers Smart Ones Three Cheese Omelet (**200 calories, 7 g fat**)

✓ CedarLane Green Chile, Cheese & Ranchero Sauce Egg White Omelette (**240 calories, 10 g fat**)

✖ STOP EATING | ✔ START EATING

✖ Denny's Hearty Breakfast Skillet (1090 calories, 85 g fat)

✖ IHOP Garden Omelette (930 calories, 76 g fat)

✖ Perkins Mediterranean Omelette (630 calories)

Choose Your Toppings and Fillings

Customize your eggs and omelets with your favorite toppings and fillings. See how many calories they are per tablespoon.

Chopped ham	27
Shredded cheddar	25
Crumbled feta	25
Ketchup	19
Cooked onion	6
Salsa	5
Cooked broccoli	3
Cooked mushrooms	3
Cooked spinach	3
Diced tomato	2

✔ Corner Bakery Café All American Egg White Scrambler (substitute chicken apple sausage for the applewood smoked bacon)

KICK START

**230 calories
10 g fat**

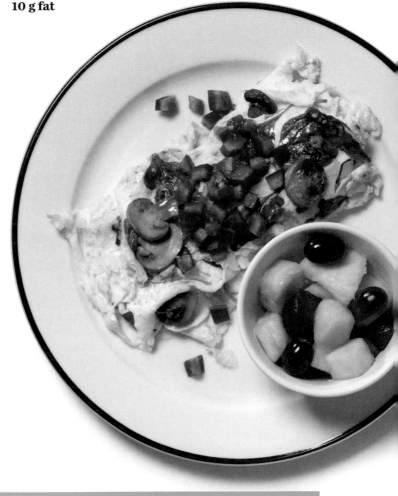

Other Good Choices

✓ Bob Evans Scrambled Eggs **(160 calories, 10 g fat)**

✓ Perkins Build Your Own Omelette with broccoli and mushrooms with a side of fruit **(305 calories, 16.5 g fat)**

✓ IHOP Simple & Fit Vegetable Omelette with fruit cup **(320 calories)**

✓ Denny's Fit Fare Veggie Skillet **(340 calories, 11 g fat)**

HASH BROWNS & HOME FRIES

❌ **STOP EATING**	✅ **START EATING**

🛒 *Packaged*

STOP EATING

✖ Idahoan Steakhouse Cheesy Hashbrown Potatoes (190 calories, 5 g fat)

✖ 1 Ore-Ida Golden Patty (140 calories, 8 g fat)

START EATING

✔ 1¼ cup Ore-Ida Shredded Hash Brown Potatoes, sautéed with no oil in a nonstick skillet

STEADY LOSS

70 calories
0 g fat

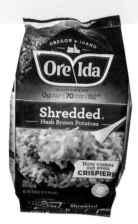

Other Good Choices

✓ ¾ cup Cascadinn Farm Premium Organic Country Style Potatoes, sautéed with no oil in a nonstick skillet **(60 calories, 0 g fat)**

✓ ⅔ cup Alexia Yukon Select Hashed Browns with Onion, Garlic & White Pepper, sautéed with no oil in a nonstick skillet **(60 calories, 0 g fat)**

✓ 1 cup Cascadian Farm Premium Organic Hash Browns, sautéed with no oil in a nonstick skillet **(60 calories, 0 g fat)**

✓ ½ cup Ore-Ida Diced Hash Brown Potatoes, sautéed with no oil in a nonstick skillet **(70 calories, 0 g fat)**

⊗ STOP EATING

✖ Hardee's Medium
Hash Rounds
(370 calories, 22 g fat)

✖ Denny's Cheddar
Cheese Hash Browns
(300 calories, 19 g fat)

✅ START EATING

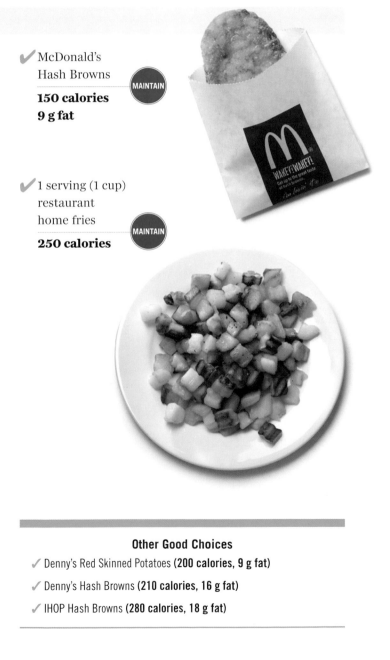

✔ McDonald's
Hash Browns

MAINTAIN

**150 calories
9 g fat**

✔ 1 serving (1 cup)
restaurant
home fries

MAINTAIN

250 calories

Other Good Choices

✓ Denny's Red Skinned Potatoes (**200 calories, 9 g fat**)

✓ Denny's Hash Browns (**210 calories, 16 g fat**)

✓ IHOP Hash Browns (**280 calories, 18 g fat**)

Breakfast Foods
YOGURT

❌ STOP EATING	✓ START EATING

🛒 *Packaged*

STOP EATING

❌ 8 oz carton Noosa Lemon Yogurt (320 calories)

❌ Yoplait Thick & Creamy Strawberry Yogurt (180 calories, 25 g sugars)

❌ Stonyfield Organic O'Soy (170 calories, 26 g sugars)

START EATING

✓ Dannon Activia Light Fat Free Vanilla Yogurt **KICK START**
60 calories
6 g sugars

✓ Yoplait Light Strawberry **KICK START**
90 calories
10 g sugars

✓ Chobani Simply 100 Blueberry Greek Yogurt **KICK START**
100 calories
8 g sugars

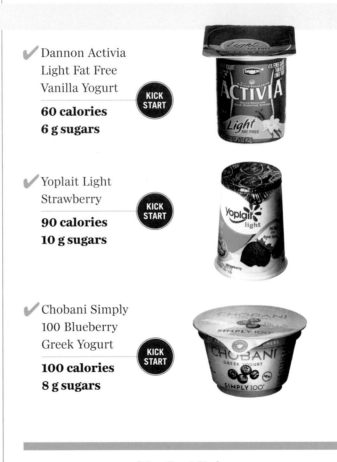

Other Good Choices

✓ Dannon Oikos Plain Nonfat Greek Yogurt (**80 calories, 6 g sugars**)

✓ Dannon Light & Fit Greek Nonfat Strawberry Yogurt (**80 calories, 6 g sugars**)

✓ Chobani Blended Lemon Greek Yogurt (**130 calories, 15 g sugars**)

✓ Fage Fruyo 0% Blueberry (**140 calories, 19 g sugars**)

✓ Chobani Fruit on the Bottom Strawberry Banana Greek Yogurt (**150 calories**)

✖ STOP EATING | ✔ START EATING

✗ *Restaurant*

✖ Au Bon Pain Blueberry
Yogurt & Wild Blueberry
Parfait (410 calories, 53 g
sugars)

✖ Starbucks Greek Yogurt
Raspberry Lemon Parfait
(310 calories)

✔ McDonald's Fruit 'n Yogurt Parfait

150 calories
23 g sugars

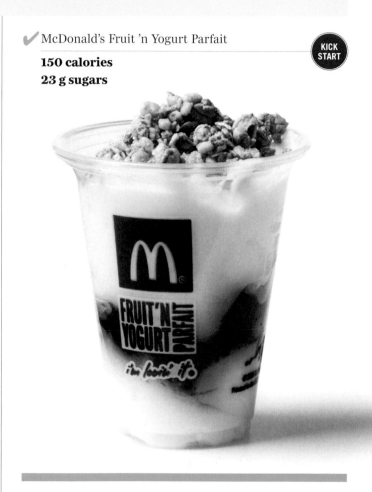

KICK
START

Other Good Choices

✓ Denny's Low Fat Yogurt **(160 calories, 25 g sugars)**

✓ Starbucks Greek Yogurt with Berries Parfait **(220 calories,
19 g sugars)**

✓ 7-Eleven Yoplait Strawberry Yogurt Parfait **(230 calories,
25 g sugars)**

Breakfast Foods
SMOOTHIES AND JUICES

⊗ **STOP EATING**	✓ **START EATING**

🏠 *Homemade*

✖ Smoothie made with ¾ cup canned coconut milk, 2 Tbsp peanut butter, 1 Tbsp honey, and 1 small banana (674 calories)

✔ Smoothie made with 1 5.2–6 oz carton (80–100 calories) 0% plain 0% Greek yogurt, 1 Tbsp peanut butter, 1 tsp honey, ½ apple (peeled, cored, and chopped), and ice

218 calories

KICK START

❌ STOP EATING | ✅ START EATING

🛒 *Packaged*

❌ 1 bottle Naked Green Machine (270 calories, 56 g sugars

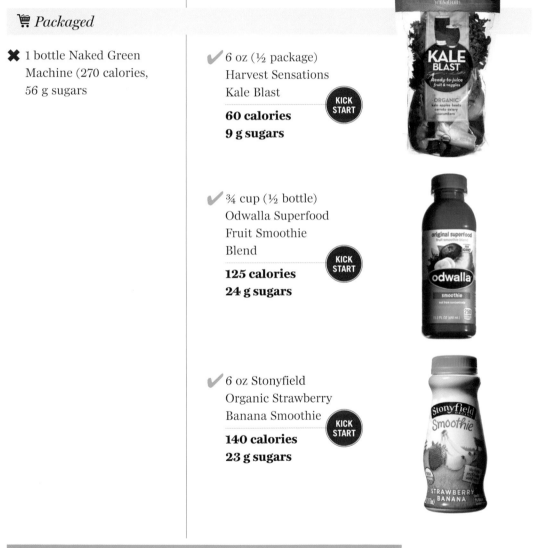

✅ 6 oz (½ package) Harvest Sensations Kale Blast

KICK START

60 calories
9 g sugars

✅ ¾ cup (½ bottle) Odwalla Superfood Fruit Smoothie Blend

KICK START

125 calories
24 g sugars

✅ 6 oz Stonyfield Organic Strawberry Banana Smoothie

KICK START

140 calories
23 g sugars

Other Good Choices

✓ 8 oz Bolthouse Farms Daily Greens **(90 calories, 19 g sugars)**

✓ 15.2 oz Bolthouse Farms Strawberry Banana Smoothie **(230 calories, 22 g sugars)**

Chapter 9
SOUPS

I could eat soup every day of the year. It warms me up, pairs perfectly with half a sandwich or a salad, and makes a meal more filling. In fact, researchers at Penn State University found that when 66 people drank soup at the beginning of a meal, they ate 20% fewer calories.[65]

There's a lot to love. Soup is convenient. It's easy to pick up canned or boxed soups or soup mixes at the market. Recipes tend to be easy to make. You can freeze individual portions to heat up when you want them. And most restaurants have at least one soup on the menu.

Some soups, though, can be high in calories. The culprits are usually cream-based or cheesy soups, such as New England clam chowder, lobster bisque, cream of mushroom, or broccoli and cheddar soup. Opt for broth-based or tomato-based soups instead, such as chicken noodle or minestrone. If you're craving a creamy soup, look for recipes or products that are marked "lower in fat" or use milk instead of cream. (In a restaurant, ask how the soup is made.)

Another possible pitfall is saturated fat from fatty meats, which are often used in soups to help make the broth richer. If your soup contains meat, look for packages made with lean meat; they may be marked "lower in fat." If you make your own, chill the soup and skim the fat that collects on the surface before you eat it.

Also, beware of toppings. Use just one packet of four saltines (64 calories) or a ½-ounce bag of oyster crackers (60 calories) instead of the whole pile. At home, swap in reduced-fat shredded cheese and swap out regular cheese on your onion soup. Make soups creamy with 0% plain Greek yogurt rather than sour cream. Add flavor to chili with vegetable garnishes such as finely chopped scallions, red onions, or chives instead of piles of cheese.

Canned soups have a particularly bad reputation for being high in sodium. We've selected the best of the bunch, but it's true that sodium can run a little high in these. Try watering them down a bit by adding an extra ½ cup of water, and also look for lower sodium versions whenever possible.

Finally, add vegetables and beans—they're filling and don't contribute an overabundance of calories. Drain canned beans first to get rid of about half the sodium! If you make or buy a soup that looks a bit skimpy on vegetables, add more! I like to keep a couple bags of frozen vegetables on hand for tossing into soup.

STOP EATING	START EATING
• Soups made with higher-fat meats such as stew beef, bacon, sausage, smoked meats, and certain cuts of pork	• Soups made with lean meats that have a lot of flavor, including turkey bacon, Canadian bacon, and smoked turkey breast
• Soups made with heavy cream or half-and-half	• Broth-based soups or soups made with lower fat dairy or nondairy milks
• Calorie-buster toppings like sour cream, grated cheese, crumbled bacon, and greasy croutons	• Chopped scallions, onions, sun-dried tomatoes, and other veggie toppings
• Soups hidden under a blanket of melted cheese	• Soups sprinkled with a strongly flavored cheese (such as Parmesan or Romano) for maximum impact on taste
• Bowls of soup, especially if oversized	• Cups of soup

CHICKEN NOODLE SOUP

❌ STOP EATING | ✅ START EATING

🛒 *Packaged*

❌ 1 package Sapporo Ichiban Japanese Style Noodles & Chicken Flavored Soup (460 calories, 2050 mg sodium)

❌ 1 block Nissin Top Ramen Chicken Flavor (380 calories, 1820 mg sodium)

✔ 1 cup soup prepared from Lipton Chicken Noodle Soup mix

(KICK START)

50 calories
540 mg sodium

✔ 1 cup (½ can) Healthy Choice Chicken Noodle Soup

(KICK START)

90 calories
390 mg sodium

✔ 1 cup (½ container) Campbell's Slow Kettle Style Roasted Chicken Noodle Soup with Herbs and White Meat Chicken

(KICK START)

100 calories
790 mg sodium

✓ START EATING

🛒 *Packaged*

✓ 1 bowl (1 container)
Annie Chun's Chinese
Chicken Soup Bowl

 MAINTAIN

300 calories
710 mg sodium

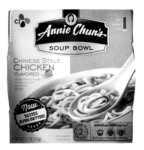

Other Good Choices

✓ 1 cup (½ can) Wolfgang Puck Organic Free Range Chicken
Noodle Soup **(90 calories, 860 mg sodium)**

✓ 1 cup (½ can) Progresso Traditional Chicken Noodle Soup
(100 calories, 690 mg sodium)

✓ 1 cup (½ can) Campbell's Chunky Chicken Noodle Soup
(110 calories, 790 mg sodium)

✓ 1 cup soup prepared from Bear Creek Country Kitchens
Chicken Noodle Soup mix **(120 calories, 650 mg sodium)**

Soups
CHILI

❌ STOP EATING | ✅ START EATING

🏠 *Homemade*

❌ 1 cup chili made with chuck beef, bacon fat, chili powder, and canned and fresh tomatoes (400 calories)

✔ 1 cup chili made with 90% lean ground beef, chili beans, chili powder, and canned and fresh tomatoes

210 calories

MAINTAIN

Choose Your Toppings

Stop and think before you sprinkle on that cheese or scoop up that sour cream. See how many calories your favorite toppings have per tablespoon.

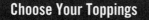

Shredded Cheddar cheese	28
Sour cream	23
Light sour cream	21
Reduced-fat cheddar cheese	20
Diced avocado	15
Plain 0% Greek yogurt	8
Diced yellow onion	4
Diced green onion	2
Diced tomato	2
Finely chopped cilantro	0

HOW TO MAKE IT

Sauté 1 pound 90% lean ground beef. Add 1 15–16 oz can chili beans, 1 Tbsp chili powder, 1 15–16 oz can tomatoes with green chiles, and 1 cup diced fresh tomato. Season to taste with salt, pepper, and additional chili powder. (Makes 6 servings)

❌ STOP EATING | ✓ START EATING

🛒 *Packaged*

❌ 1 cup (½ container)
Zeigler Chili con Carne
(670 calories, 57 g fat)

❌ 1 cup (½ can) Wolf
Brand Chili No Beans
(400 calories, 29 g fat)

✓ 1 pouch (½ package)
Tabatchnick
Vegetarian Chili **KICK START**

**180 calories
3.5 g fat**

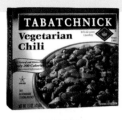

✓ 1 cup (½ can)
Hormel Turkey Chili
No Beans **KICK START**

**190 calories
3 g fat**

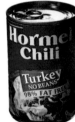

Other Good Choices

✓ 1 cup (½ can) Wolf Brand Chili Lean Beef No Beans **(220 calories, 6 g fat)**

✓ 1 cup (½ can) Campbell's Chunky Beef & Bean Roadhouse Chili **(220 calories, 6 g fat)**

✓ 1 cup (½ can) Amy's Organic Medium Chili **(280 calories, 9 g fat)**

🍴 *Restaurant*

❌ 1 bowl Applebee's Chili
(410 calories,
24 g fat)

❌ 1 cup Corner Bakery
Café Big Al's Chili
(380 calories, 17 g fat)

✓ Small Wendy's Rich
and Meaty Chili **STEADY LOSS**

**170 calories
5 g fat**

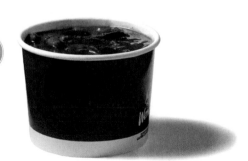

Other Good Choices

✓ 1 cup Chili's Terlingua Chili **(200 calories, 14 g fat)**

✓ Regular Cosi Southwest Corn & Turkey Chili **(290 calories, 14 g fat)**

❌ STOP EATING | ✅ START EATING

🛒 *Packaged*

❌ 1 cup (½ container) Legal Sea Foods refrigerated New England Clam Chowder (290 calories, 20 g fat)

✔ 1 cup (½ can) Bar Harbor Manahattan Style Clam Chowder

KICK START

70 calories
0.5 g fat

✔ 1 cup (½ can) Progresso Traditional New England Clam Chowder

MAINTAIN

180 calories
8 g fat

SUPER SWITCH
Switch to 1 cup Progresso 99% Fat Free New England Clam Chowder and drop another 60 calories and 5 g fat!

Other Good Choices

✓ 1 cup (½ can) Progresso Traditional Manhattan Clam Chowder
(100 calories, 2 g fat)

✓ 1 cup (½ can) Campbell's Chunky Manhattan Clam Chowder
(120 calories, 3 g fat)

✓ 1 cup (½ can) Campbell's Healthy Request New England Chowder
(130 calories, 3 g fat)

⊗ STOP EATING | ⊘ START EATING

✖ TGI Friday's New
England Clam Chowder
(500 calories, 30 g fat)

✖ 1 cup Panera New
England Clam Chowder
(480 calories, 42 g fat)

✔ 1 cup Denny's
Clam
Chowder

MAINTAIN

**200 calories
9 g fat**

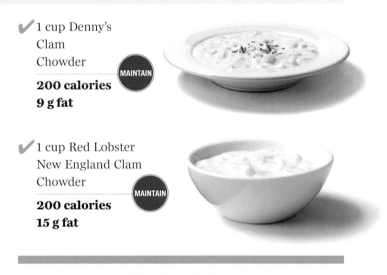

✔ 1 cup Red Lobster
New England Clam
Chowder

MAINTAIN

**200 calories
15 g fat**

Other Good Choices

✓ 1 cup Legal Sea Foods Lite Clam Chowder (**76 calories**)

✓ 1 cup Joe's Crab Shack New England Clam Chowder (**250 calories,
13 g fat**)

Soups
TOMATO SOUP

❌ STOP EATING	✅ START EATING

🛒 *Packaged*

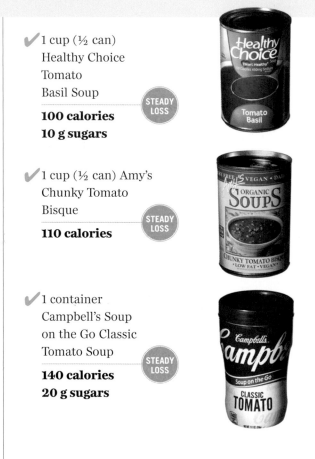

STOP EATING

❌ 1 container Campbell's Soup on the Go Creamy Tomato Soup (220 calories, 21 g sugars)

❌ 1 cup (½ can) Campbell's Tomato Roasted Garlic Bacon Bisque (210 calories, 22 g sugars)

START EATING

✓ 1 cup (½ can) Healthy Choice Tomato Basil Soup
STEADY LOSS
100 calories
10 g sugars

✓ 1 cup (½ can) Amy's Chunky Tomato Bisque
STEADY LOSS
110 calories

✓ 1 container Campbell's Soup on the Go Classic Tomato Soup
STEADY LOSS
140 calories
20 g sugars

Other Good Choices

✓ 1 cup (½ can) Progresso Heart Healthy Tomato with Parmesan **(80 calories, 9 g sugars)**

✓ 1 cup (¼ carton) Imagine Organic Creamy Tomato Soup **(80 calories, 9 g sugars)**

✓ 1 cup (½ can) Amy's Organic Cream of Tomato Soup **(110 calories, 13 g sugars)**

✓ 1 cup (½ carton) Progresso Artisan Tomato and Roasted Red Pepper Soup **(150 calories, 11 g sugar)**

❌ STOP EATING | ✓ START EATING

❌ 1 cup Panera Vegetarian Creamy Tomato Soup (330 calories, 23 g fat)

❌ TGI Friday's Tomato Basil Soup (300 calories, 24 g fat)

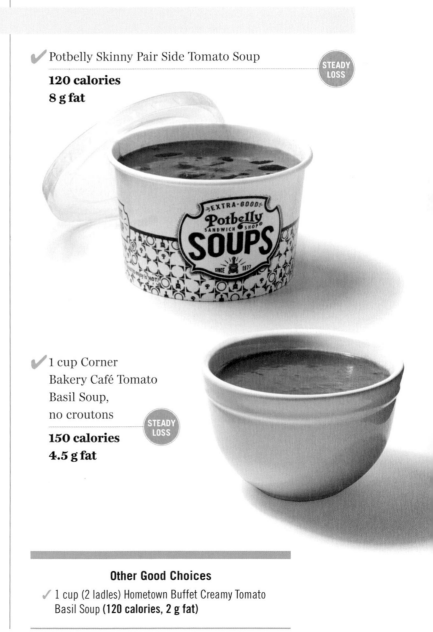

✓ Potbelly Skinny Pair Side Tomato Soup

120 calories
8 g fat

STEADY LOSS

✓ 1 cup Corner Bakery Café Tomato Basil Soup, no croutons

150 calories
4.5 g fat

STEADY LOSS

Other Good Choices

✓ 1 cup (2 ladles) Hometown Buffet Creamy Tomato Basil Soup (**120 calories, 2 g fat**)

Soups

VEGETABLE AND MINESTRONE SOUPS

❌ **STOP EATING**	✅ **START EATING**

🛒 *Packaged*

❌ 1 cup (½ can) Amy's Organic Fire Roasted Southwestern Vegetable Soup (140 calories)

❌ 1 cup (½ can) Colavita Minestrone Soup (130 calories)

✅ 1 cup (½ can) Health Valley No Salt Added Minestrone **KICK START**

90 calories
50 mg sodium

✅ 1 cup (½ can) Campbell's Chunky Savory Vegetable Soup **KICK START**

100 calories

✅ 1 cup (½ can) Progresso Vegetable Classics Minestrone **KICK START**

100 calories
4 g fiber

Other Good Choices

✓ 1 cup (½ can) Progresso Light Italian-Style Vegetable Soup **(70 calories, 4 g fiber)**

✓ 1 cup (½ can) Amy's Organic Low Fat Minestrone **(90 calories)**

✓ 1 cup (½ can) Progresso Rich & Hearty Slow Cooked Vegetable Beef Soup **(120 calories)**

✓ 1 cup (½ can) Wolfgang Puck Organic Classic Minestrone **(120 calories)**

✕ STOP EATING | ✓ START EATING

✗ *Restaurant*

✕ 1 order Macaroni Grill Minestrone Soup (160 calories)

✕ 1 cup Souplantation Vegetarian Harvest Soup (130 calories, 8 g fat)

✓ 1 cup Panera Low-Fat Vegetarian Garden Vegetable Soup with Pesto **KICK START**

90 calories

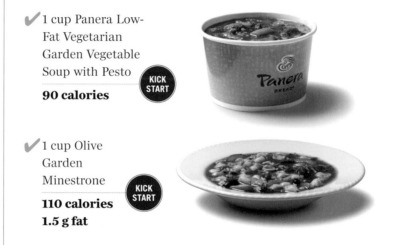

✓ 1 cup Olive Garden Minestrone **KICK START**

**110 calories
1.5 g fat**

Other Good Choices

✓ Small (1 cup) Au Bon Pain Vegetarian Minestrone **(80 calories)**

✓ 1 cup Souplantation Vegetable Medley Soup **(90 calories, 1 g fat)**

Soups
CREAM SOUPS

⊗ STOP EATING	⊘ START EATING

🛒 *Packaged*

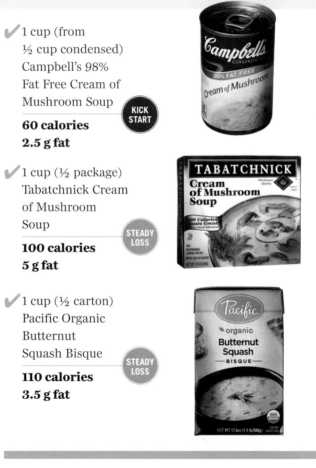

STOP EATING

✖ 1 cup (½ can) Campbell's Slow Kettle Style Creamy Broccoli Cheddar Bisque (180 calories, 13 g fat)

✖ 1 cup (½ can) Wolfgang Puck Signature Butternut Squash Soup (150 calories, 8 g fat)

✖ 1 cup (¼ carton) Imagine Loaded Baked Potato Soup (120 calories, 5 g fat)

START EATING

✔ 1 cup (from ½ cup condensed) Campbell's 98% Fat Free Cream of Mushroom Soup — **KICK START**
60 calories
2.5 g fat

✔ 1 cup (½ package) Tabatchnick Cream of Mushroom Soup — **STEADY LOSS**
100 calories
5 g fat

✔ 1 cup (½ carton) Pacific Organic Butternut Squash Bisque — **STEADY LOSS**
110 calories
3.5 g fat

Other Good Choices

✓ 1 cup (¼ carton) Imagine Light in Sodium Creamy Garden Broccoli Soup **(70 calories, 1.5 g fat)**

✓ 1 cup (½ can) Health Valley Organic Cream of Mushroom Soup **(90 calories, 2 g fat)**

✓ 1 cup (from ½ cup condensed) Campbell's Cream of Potato Soup **(90 calories, 2 g fat)**

❌ STOP EATING

✗ *Restaurant*

❌ Ruby Tuesday Broccoli and Cheese Soup (325 calories, 22 g fat)

❌ Longhorn Steakhouse Mushroom Truffle Bisque (280 calories, 19 g fat)

❌ 1 cup Red Lobster Creamy Potato Bacon Soup (250 calories, 18 g fat)

✔ START EATING

✔ 1 cup Panera Broccoli Cheddar Soup

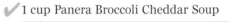

MAINTAIN

220 calories
14 g fat

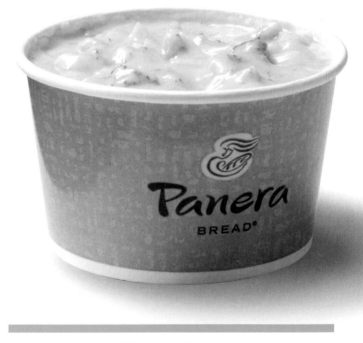

Other Good Choices

✓ 1 cup Jersey Mike's Broccoli Cheese with Florets **(140 calories, 9 g fat)**

✓ 1 cup Jersey Mike's Cream of Potato **(180 calories, 8 g fat)**

BARLEY, LENTIL, AND PEA SOUPS

❌ STOP EATING | ✓ START EATING

🛒 *Packaged*

STOP EATING

❌ 1 container Spice Hunter Split Pea Vegetarian Soup (190 calories)

❌ 1 cup (½ can) Progresso Vegetable Classics Lentil Soup (160 calories)

❌ 1 cup (prepared from ¼ package) Alessi Lenticchie Sicilian Lentil Soup (150 calories)

START EATING

✓ 1 cup (½ can) Amy's Organic Split Pea Soup   **KICK START**

100 calories 0 g fat

✓ 1 cup (½ bowl) Healthy Choice Hearty Vegetable Barley   **STEADY LOSS**

140 calories

✓ 1 cup (½ can) Campbell's Chunky Hearty Beef Barley Soup   **STEADY LOSS**

140 calories

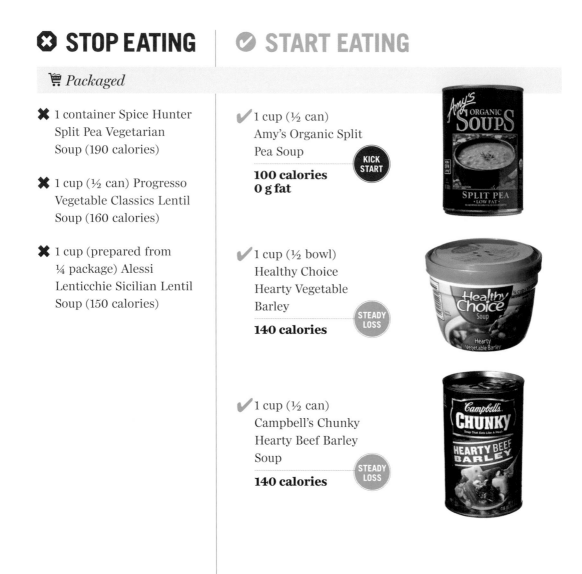

✅ START EATING

🛒 *Packaged*

✔ 1 cup (½ can) Progresso Vegetable Classics 99% Fat Free Lentil Soup
STEADY LOSS
140 calories
1.5 g fat

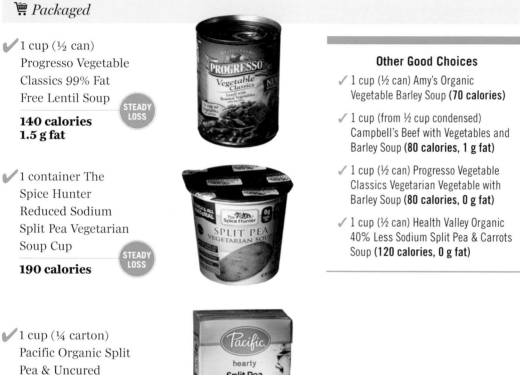

✔ 1 container The Spice Hunter Reduced Sodium Split Pea Vegetarian Soup Cup
STEADY LOSS
190 calories

✔ 1 cup (¼ carton) Pacific Organic Split Pea & Uncured Ham Soup
STEADY LOSS
160 calories

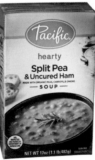

Other Good Choices

✓ 1 cup (½ can) Amy's Organic Vegetable Barley Soup (**70 calories**)

✓ 1 cup (from ½ cup condensed) Campbell's Beef with Vegetables and Barley Soup (**80 calories, 1 g fat**)

✓ 1 cup (½ can) Progresso Vegetable Classics Vegetarian Vegetable with Barley Soup (**80 calories, 0 g fat**)

✓ 1 cup (½ can) Health Valley Organic 40% Less Sodium Split Pea & Carrots Soup (**120 calories, 0 g fat**)

Soups
FRENCH ONION SOUP

❌ **STOP EATING**	✅ **START EATING**

🏠 *Homemade*

❌ French onion soup made with 1 cup beef broth, 1 cup onions, 1 slice bread, and 2 Tbsp Gruyere cheese (256 calories, 1100 mg sodium)

✔ French onion soup made with Swanson Beef Broth, onions, Melba toast, and grated Parmesan cheese

KICK START

132 calories

HOW TO MAKE IT

Sauté 4 cups onions in 1 tsp oil until soft. Heat with 4 cups Swanson Beef Broth. Dish into 4 bowls. Top with 1 piece Melba toast and 1 Tbsp grated Parmesan cheese. (Makes 4 servings)

✖ STOP EATING | ✔ START EATING

🛒 *Packaged*

✖ 1 cup soup made from ¼ cup Frontier Soups Chicago Bistro French Onion Soup Mix (220 calories, 790 mg sodium)

✔ 1 cup Tabatchnick Frenchman's Onion Soup

KICK START

60 calories
500 mg sodium

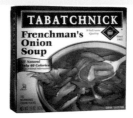

Other Good Choices

✓ 1 cup (¼ container) Pacific Organic French Onion Soup **(30 calories)**

✓ 1 cup (½ can) Progresso Vegetable Classics French Onion Soup **(50 calories)**

✓ 1 cup (from ½ cup condensed) Campbell's French Onion Soup **(70 calories)**

🍴 *Restaurant*

✖ 1 bowl Longhorn Steakhouse French Onion Soup (380 calories)

✖ 1 bowl Applebee's French Onion Soup (370 calories, 23 g fat)

✔ 1 cup Panera Bistro French Onion Soup

KICK START

200 calories

✔ 1 bowl TGI Friday's French Onion Soup

STEADY LOSS

360 calories

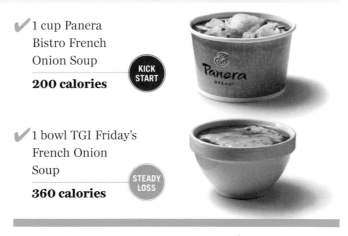

Other Good Choice

✓ 1 cup Au Bon Pain French Onion Soup **(70 calories)**

Chapter 10
SALADS

When I'm in the mood for a full plate of food, I have a salad. I can pile up the lettuce and veggies knowing that they don't have many calories. Generally if the vegetable is in its natural state—no dressing or sauce—it's almost a freebie!

The number one caution with salads is: Pay attention to the dressing. In researching this book, I came across a lot of restaurant websites that list the calories and nutrition in their salads, with and without dressing. What an eye-opener! Salad dressing can add hundreds of calories to a pretty innocent-sounding salad. Those little packets have too much dressing (of course it's hard not to use it all), and the dressing tends to be packed with calories. Throughout this chapter, I've sprinkled additional information on dressings, and you'll also find specific dressing suggestions among some of the good choices.

But many of the salads I recommend don't include dressing at all. I find that just the addition of a few flavorful ingredients like olives or artichokes can add enough oomph that dressing isn't even needed. In other cases, just a few dashes of vinegar (try red wine vinegar or balsamic vinegar) or a squeeze of lemon juice does the trick. At home, you can give your salad a few sprays of oil from a Misto or pressurized can, toss it, and then sprinkle with vinegar and fresh herbs. The oil softens the sharpness of the vinegar. If you really miss having a creamy dressing, try my secret: 0% plain Greek yogurt blended with some fresh herbs!

My second caution pertains to toppings. Some salad toppings should come with warning signs because they're so high in fat and calories and have very little that is good for health or weight loss. I'm talking to you, fried croutons, fried wonton noodles, crumbled bacon, shredded or crumbled cheese, and candied nuts. Instead, I enjoy a bit of avocado or nuts and seeds for MUFAs.

When I have a salad as my meal, it has to have protein to be balanced and satisfying. Nothing fancy here, maybe grilled chicken breast, lean steak, or salmon. My tuna is always packed in water, not oil, and I like to keep a couple of pouches handy for a quick addition to a garden salad.

Last, an amazing find: Dozens of companies are getting into the ready-made green salad business. I may never buy a head of lettuce again! I love that my market has dozens of choices that contain nutrition-packed greens like kale and spinach. Some of these have protein, some have toppings and dressing, and some are just plain veggies. Pay close attention to the wording on packaged salads. A salad blend tends to be just greens. A salad kit also has toppings and dressing. Kits have more calories so you can't really swap one for the other. I've recommended several of these to get you started.

STOP EATING	START EATING
• Sugary, oily, or fattening dressings in big portions, with more calories than the salad itself	• Dressings with a little good fat and fewer calories, sprinkled on, or vinegar plus a few sprays of flavorful oil
• Salads hiding under calorie-rich toppings such as croutons, fried wonton noodles, bacon, candied nuts, and grated cheese	• A couple teaspoons of crunchy, crispy toppings, such as chopped nuts, chia seeds, and toasted garbanzo beans (they're pretty popular and widely available these days), tossed well to spread throughout the salad
• Protein from breaded and fried chicken or fish, higher-fat steak, and large portions of deli meats and cheeses	• Protein from grilled chicken breast, salmon, or lean beef, or a modest portion of lean deli meats
• Low-flavor, low-fiber, low-nutrition greens such as iceberg lettuce	• Dark green, purple, and other colorful salad greens for more vitamin C, nutrients, and healthful plant compounds
• Greasy or fatty deli salads such as potato salad, pasta salad, and coleslaw	• Produce department salad kits or DIY salads, where you control the dressing

Salads
CHICKEN CAESAR SALADS

⊗ STOP EATING	⊘ START EATING

🏠 Homemade

✖ Chicken Caesar salad made with 3.5 oz (⅓ bag) Dole Ultimate Caesar Salad Kit and 3 oz grilled chicken breast (310 calories)

✔ Chicken Caesar salad made with 3.5 oz (⅓ bag) Fresh Express CaesarLite Kit and 3 oz grilled chicken breast

230 calories

KICK START

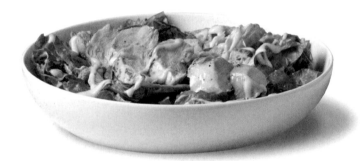

🛒 Packaged

✖ Ready Pac Bistro Bowl Organic Caesar Salad with Chicken (270 calories, 22 g fat)

✖ Fresh Express Chicken Caesar (270 calories, 21 g fat)

✔ Ready Pac Bistro Bowl Caesar Lite Salad with chicken

KICK START

180 calories
10 g fat

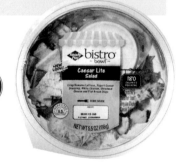

Other Good Choices

✓ Dole Light Caesar Salad Kit **(90 calories, 6 g fat)**

✓ Taylor Farms Chicken Caesar Salad **(200 calories, 12 g fat)**

✓ Ready Pac Bistro Bowl Chicken Caesar Salad **(230 calories, 16 g fat)**

✖ STOP EATING | ✔ START EATING

✖ Cheesecake Factory Small Salad Caesar with Chicken (980 calories)

✖ Red Lobster Classic Caesar with Chicken (660 calories, 53 g fat)

✖ Wendy's Spicy Chicken Caesar, with croutons, no dressing (570 calories, 1290 mg sodium)

✔ Au Bon Pain Chicken Caesar Asiago, no dressing

STEADY LOSS

250 calories
530 mg sodium

✔ Applebee's lunch menu Grilled Chicken Caesar Salad, no dressing

STEADY LOSS

295 calories
17 g fat

Other Good Choice

✓ TGI Friday's lunch menu Balsamic-Glazed Chicken Caesar Salad **(350 calories)**

Salads
ASIAN CHICKEN SALADS

❌ STOP EATING | ✅ START EATING

🛒 *Packaged*

✖ 3.5 oz (⅓ bag) Taylor Farms Asian Chopped Salad Kit, with dressing plus 3 oz grilled chicken breast (300 calories)

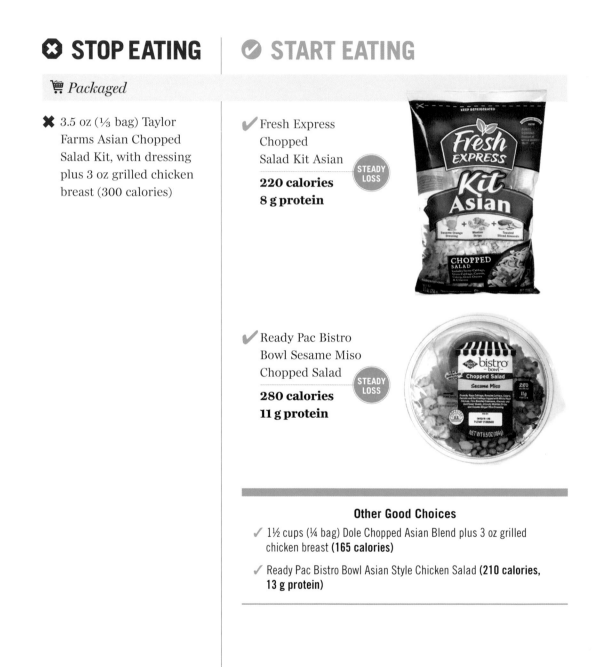

✔ Fresh Express Chopped Salad Kit Asian

220 calories
8 g protein

STEADY LOSS

✔ Ready Pac Bistro Bowl Sesame Miso Chopped Salad

280 calories
11 g protein

STEADY LOSS

Other Good Choices

✓ 1½ cups (¼ bag) Dole Chopped Asian Blend plus 3 oz grilled chicken breast **(165 calories)**

✓ Ready Pac Bistro Bowl Asian Style Chicken Salad **(210 calories, 13 g protein)**

✖ STOP EATING | ✔ START EATING

✗ *Restaurant*

✖ Applebee's Oriental
Grilled Chicken Salad
(1290 calories, 82 g fat)

✖ Cheesecake Factory
Chinese Chicken Salad
(960 calories)

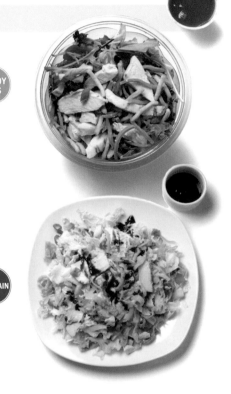

✔ Cosi Shanghai
Chicken Salad **STEADY LOSS**

265 calories
18 g protein

✔ Half size California
Pizza Kitchen
Chinese Chicken
Salad **MAINTAIN**

395 calories
18 g fat

Other Good Choices

✓ Half size Panera Asian Sesame Chicken Salad, no dressing
(200 calories, 16 g protein)

✓ Wendy's Asian Cashew Chicken Salad, with dressing **(335 calories,
35 g protein)**

✓ Au Bon Pain Thai Peanut Chicken Salad **(350 calories, 13 g fat)**

Salads
WALDORF AND APPLE SALADS

❌ STOP EATING | ✅ START EATING

🏠 *Homemade*

✖ Waldorf salad made with 2 cups lettuce, ½ cup chopped apple, 2 Tbsp chopped walnuts, 2 Tbsp chopped celery, and 1 Tbsp mayonnaise (245 calories)

✔ Waldorf salad made with 2 cups lettuce, 1 cup chopped apple, 1 Tbsp chopped walnuts, 2 Tbsp chopped celery, and 1 Tbsp 0% plain Greek yogurt

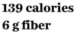

139 calories
6 g fiber

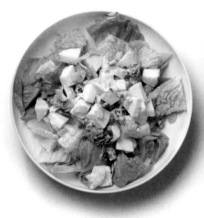

🛒 *Packaged*

✔ Ready Pac Bistro Bowl Apple Bleu Pecan Salad, with dressing

MAINTAIN

230 calories

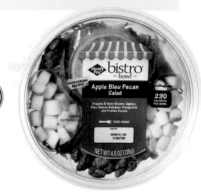

❌ STOP EATING | ✅ START EATING

❌ Potbelly Uptown Salad, with Potbelly Vinaigrette (624 calories, 42 g fat)

❌ Half size California Pizza Kitchen Waldorf Chicken Salad, with dressing (610 calories, 44 g fat)

❌ Burger King Chicken Apple & Cranberry Garden Fresh Salad with dressing (480 calories, 34 g sugars)

✔ Wendy's Apple Pecan Chicken Salad, no dressing or toppings

MAINTAIN

350 calories
17 g sugars

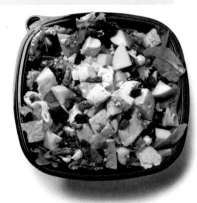

✔ Denny's Cranberry Apple Chicken Salad, with balsamic vinaigrette

MAINTAIN

360 calories
9 g fat

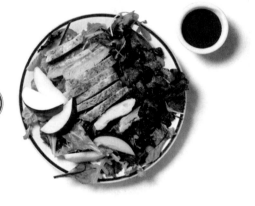

Other Good Choices

✓ 1 cup Souplantation Nutty Waldorf Salad (**180 calories, 6 g fat**)

✓ Half size Panera Fuji Apple Chicken Salad, no dressing (**280 calories, 11 g sugar**)

✓ Au Bon Pain Wheatberry Waldorf Salad Petit Plate (**310 calories, 14 g fat**)

Salads
CHEF'S SALADS AND COBB SALADS

❌ STOP EATING | ✅ START EATING

🏠 *Homemade*

❌ Chef's salad made with 2 oz each turkey, ham, and American cheese, 1 hard-boiled egg, 2 cups lettuce or mixed greens, 4 tomato wedges, and ¼ cup ranch dressing (688 calories)

✔ Chef's salad made with 1 oz each turkey, ham, and reduced-fat Swiss cheese, 2 hard-boiled egg whites, 2 cups lettuce or mixed greens, 8 tomato wedges, and 2 Tbsp reduced-fat ranch dressing

310 calories

KICK START

Choose Your Protein

Build a lighter chef's salad by varying which proteins you add. See how many calories are in common options.

1 oz American cheese	94
1 oz reduced-fat Swiss cheese	91
1 hard-boiled egg	78
1 strip bacon	54
1 oz turkey breast	42
1 oz deli ham	37
2 hard-boiled egg whites	34

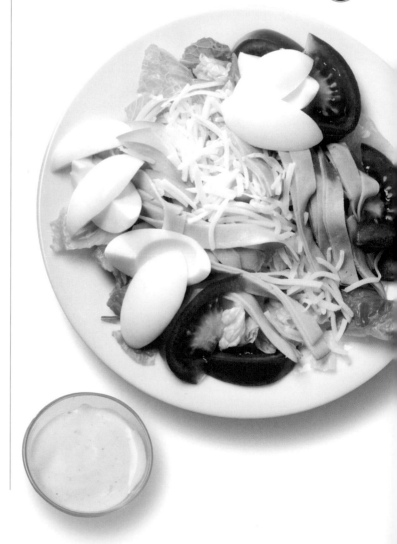

❌ STOP EATING | ✅ START EATING

✅ START EATING

🍴 *Restaurant*

❌ Panera Chicken Cobb with Avocado, with BBQ ranch dressing (800 calories, 62 g fat)

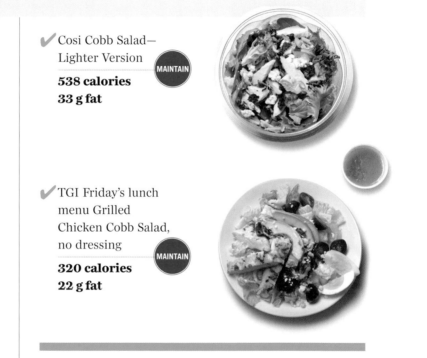

✔ Cosi Cobb Salad— Lighter Version **MAINTAIN**

538 calories
33 g fat

✔ TGI Friday's lunch menu Grilled Chicken Cobb Salad, no dressing **MAINTAIN**

320 calories
22 g fat

Other Good Choices

✓ Bob Evans Cobb Salad no dressing (**300 calories, 17 g fat**)

✓ Jersey Mike's Chef Salad, with light Italian dressing (**335 calories**)

✓ Burger King Chicken BLT Garden Fresh Salad with TENDERGRILL, with dressing (**440 calories**)

GREEK AND SPINACH SALADS

❌ STOP EATING | ✅ START EATING

🏠 *Homemade*

❌ Greek salad made from
2 cups lettuce, ¼ cup
crumbled feta cheese,
and ¼ cup croutons,
5 olives, 2 stuffed grape
leaves, and ¼ cup
vinaigrette (470 calories,
35 g fat)

✔ Greek salad made from 2 cups (½ bag) Dole
Mediterranean Blend, ¼ cup crumbled reduced-fat
feta cheese, and 2 Tbsp light Italian dressing

KICK START

125 calories
7.5 g fat

❌ STOP EATING | ✅ START EATING

🛒 Packaged

❌ Taylor Farms Spinach
Harvest Salad
(340 calories)

❌ Ready Pac Bistro Bowl
Spinach Dijon Salad
(280 calories)

❌ Earthbound Farm
Spinach Quinoa
Powermeal Bowl
(210 calories)

✅ ⅓ package Dole Spinach
Cherry Almond Bleu Salad
Kit, plus 1 cup
extra spinach **STEADY LOSS**

190 calories

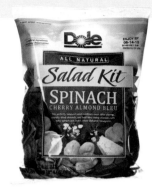

Other Good Choices

✓ 3.5 oz container Earthbound Farm California Blend Dried
Blueberries and Almonds with Organic Baby Spinach, no dressing
(90 calories)

✓ 2 cups (½ bag) Ready Pac Baby Spinach Complete Salad Kit
(140 calories)

✓ 3.5 oz (⅓ package) Dole Endless Summer Salad Kit **(150 calories,
4 g sugars)**

🍴 Restaurant

❌ Applebee's seasonal
Berry and Spinach Salad
(620 calories)

❌ Diner Greek salad, with
dressing (437 calories)

❌ 2 cups Souplantation
Sonoma Spinach Salad
with Honey Dijon
Vinaigrette (420 calories)

✅ Panera Greek Salad,
no dressing **MAINTAIN**

370 calories

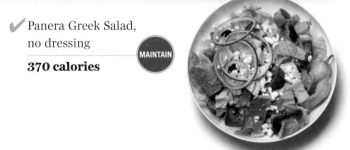

Other Good Choices

✓ Potbelly Mediterranean Salad, no dressing **(257 calories)**

✓ Cosi Greek Salad—Taste Two, with dressing **(266 calories)**

✓ Applebee's lunch menu Grilled Shrimp 'N Spinach Salad
(270 calories)

Salads
PASTA AND POTATO SALADS

❌ **STOP EATING**	✅ **START EATING**

🏠 *Homemade*

❌ Potato salad made with ½ cup cooked potatoes, 2 Tbsp mayonnaise, and 1 Tbsp pickle relish (285 calories, 28 g fat)

✅ Potato salad made with ½ cup cooked potatoes, 1 tsp olive oil, 2 tsp lemon juice, and salt and pepper to taste

STEADY LOSS

114 calories
5 g fat

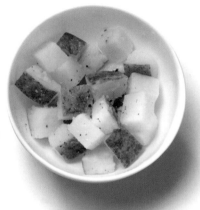

🛒 *Packaged*

❌ 1 cup prepared from ¼ package Betty Crocker Ranch & Bacon Suddenly Pasta Salad, made with mayonnaise (350 calories, 21 g fat)

✅ ½ cup (⅓ can) READ German Potato Salad

STEADY LOSS

120 calories
3 g fat

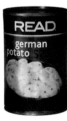

✅ 1 cup salad prepared from ¼ package Betty Crocker Ranch & Bacon Suddenly Pasta Salad, made with light mayonnaise

MAINTAIN

241 calories
8.5 g fat

SUPER SWITCH
Switch to making it with 0% plain Greek yogurt and drop another 54 calories

❌ STOP EATING | ✅ START EATING

❌ Potbelly Macaroni Salad
(450 calories, 26 g fat)

❌ ½ cup deli rotelli pasta
salad made with pasta,
olives, peppers, carrots,
and Italian dressing
(390 calories, 23 g fat)

❌ Potbelly Potato Salad
(330 calories, 25 g fat)

✔ ½ cup deli California-style pasta salad
with pasta, fresh veggies, and light vinaigrette

230 calories
3.5 g fat

MAINTAIN

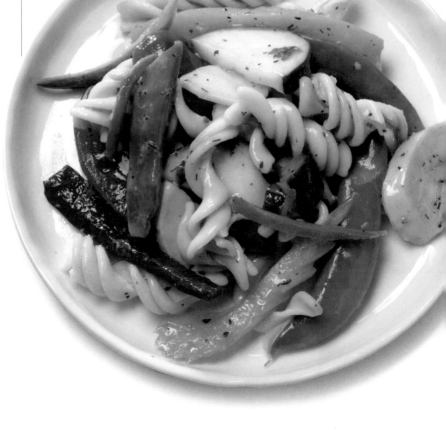

Other Good Choices

✓ ½ cup Souplantation
Mediterranean
Bistro Potato Salad
(115 calories, 5.5 g fat)

✓ Corner Bakery Café
Cavatappi Pasta Salad
(160 calories, 5 g fat)

✓ McAlister's Deli Pasta
Salad **(160 calories,
9 g fat)**

Salads
BEAN AND SIDE SALADS

⊗ STOP EATING | ✓ START EATING

🏠 *Homemade*

✖ Bean salad made with chickpeas, kidney beans, green beans, olive oil, salt, pepper, and herbs to taste (215 calories, 16 g fat)

✔ Bean salad made with chickpeas, kidney beans, green beans, and light Italian dressing

STEADY LOSS

116 calories
3.5 g fat

HOW TO MAKE IT

Mix together ½ cup each canned chickpeas and kidney beans, drained; 1 cup cooked green beans; and 4 Tbsp light Italian dressing. (Makes 4 servings)

❌ STOP EATING | ✅ START EATING

🛒 *Packaged*

❌ ½ cup Jake & Amos Four Bean Salad (140 calories, 28 g sugars)

❌ ½ cup Paisley Farm Four-Bean Salad (125 calories, 22 g sugars)

✔️ 1 ½ cups (about ½ package) Cut'N Clean Greens SuperKALE Salad slaw plus 1 Tbsp light mayonnaise

KICK START

67 calories
2.5 g fat

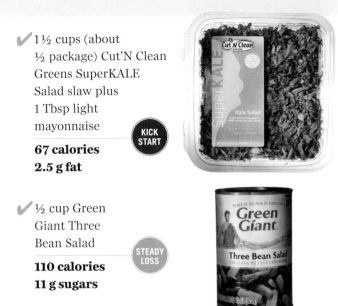

✔️ ½ cup Green Giant Three Bean Salad

STEADY LOSS

110 calories
11 g sugars

Other Good Choice
✓ ½ cup (⅕ can) READ 3 Bean Salad **(60 calories, 0 g fat)**

🍴 *Restaurant*

❌ ½ cup deli coleslaw (270 calories)

❌ Chili's Side House Salad, no dressing (150 calories)

✔️ Wendy's Garden Side Salad, no dressing or croutons

KICK START

25 calories

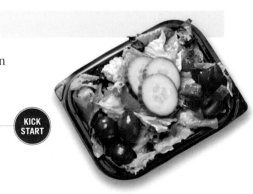

Other Good Choices
✓ Wendy's Caesar Side Salad, no dressing or croutons **(60 calories)**

✓ Arby's Chopped Side Salad with 1 packet Light Italian dressing **(90 calories)**

Chapter 11
SANDWICHES

I could eat a sandwich every day for the rest of my life. Love 'em. Love the taste, the mouthfeel, the satiety. And I love their portability. I can have a sandwich anywhere—at home, in my car (bad habit), at my desk (another bad habit), or sitting at a restaurant. What I don't like is that those bread calories add up pretty quickly, especially if I stray from standard sliced bread. See the chart at right to compare calories in different breads. And watch the calories in wraps and tortillas (chart at right). Just because they're flat doesn't mean they're low in calories.

There are so many ways to make a really satisfying sandwich from protein plus veggies plus a spread. Let's talk protein first. Lean, lean, lean—you don't want to waste precious calories on the fats in pork bacon, fatty steak, or fried chicken. This chapter profiles lots of lean choices, including turkey breast, chicken breast, roast beef, and tuna, plus a couple of higher-fat meatless options such as cheese (delivers calcium, but watch the fat and calories!) and nut butters. Nut butters, and also avocado, are overflowing with healthy MUFAs . . . and calories.

Veggies are easy. You can add the obvious lettuce and tomato, switch to fresh or roasted peppers, add darker greens such as kale or spinach, or toss in some leftover grilled vegetables. Subway and other sub sandwich shops are pretty generous with the veggies, so pile them on for barely any calories, more flavor and crunch, and no extra cost! Marinated vegetables are typically bathed in oil, so if you have them at home, give them a quick rinse and dry before adding them to your sandwich.

Finally, compare calories in different spreads (page 56). Mustard is almost a freebie and comes in different flavors and textures. Mayo and "salad dressing" (e.g., Miracle Whip) are nearly all oil, with lots of calories. Light versions are somewhat lower in calories. Sometimes I use hummus or guacamole as my spread, but I use a light hand so that I don't blow calories out of the water.

CHOOSE YOUR BREAD OR ROLL

See how many calories are in common sandwich breads and rolls.

Focaccia bread (4 oz) 282

Pepperidge Farm Farmhouse Hearty White (2 slices)............................ 220

Ciabatta roll (2½ oz) 210

Pretzel roll (2½ oz).. 180

Whole wheat pita (6 inch) 170

Kaiser roll (2 oz).. 167

Thinly sliced Italian bread (2 slices) 153

Arnold Stone Ground 100% Whole Wheat Bread (2 slices)................... 130

Pepperidge Farm Very Thin 100% Whole Wheat (2 slices)..................... 73

CHOOSE YOUR SANDWICH WRAP

See how many calories are in common sandwich wraps.

12-inch burrito wrap tortilla 300

Mission Original Wrap 210

Rice paper wrap 200

La Tortilla Factory Traditional Sonoma Organic Wrap 180

7-inch flour tortilla.. 147

Flatout 100% Whole Wheat 100

Tumaro's Low-in-Carb Multigrain Wrap 60

STOP EATING	START EATING
• Big rolls, large bagels, and thick slices of bread	• Sandwich thins, mini bagels, and thin-sliced breads
• Whole wrap sandwiches on big (10-inch) tortillas	• Half of a wrap sandwich (save or share the other half) or a homemade wrap on a 7-inch standard-size tortilla
• Highly marbled roast beef, fried chicken, thick slices of cheese, and other higher-fat proteins	• Lean roast beef, turkey, and ham, limited to 3 to 4 ounces—3 to 4 slices or more if thin sliced or shaved—per sandwich
• Huge slatherings of peanut or almond butter	• A modest schmear of nut butter, mixed with a protein-rich, lower-fat partner like silken tofu or part-skim ricotta
• Liberal uses of regular mayo	• A thin layer (about 2 teaspoons) of light mayo, mustard, or other healthy spread
• Oily grilled or roasted vegetables	• Marinated vegetables (drained and rinsed if oil-packed), home-roasted veggies with just a couple sprays of oil, or fresh veggies

Sandwiches
TURKEY SANDWICHES

❌ STOP EATING | ### ✅ START EATING

🏠 *Homemade*

❌ Turkey sandwich made with 4 oz foccacia, 5 oz turkey breast, 2 Tbsp mayonnaise, and 2 slices provolone cheese (806 calories)

✔ Turkey sandwich made with 2½ oz pretzel roll, 3 oz turkey breast, lettuce, tomato, and mustard

289 calories

KICK START

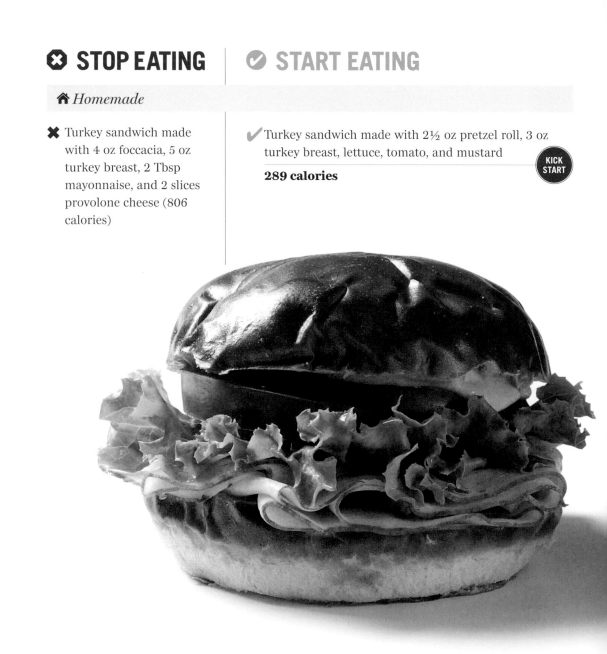

❌ STOP EATING | ✅ START EATING

❌ Panera Smokehouse Turkey Panini on Three Cheese Bread (720 calories, 2590 mg sodium)

❌ Arby's Roast Turkey & Swiss Sandwich (700 calories, 1760 mg sodium)

✔ Einstein Bros. Bagels Roasted Turkey Sandwich

STEADY LOSS

380 calories
870 mg sodium

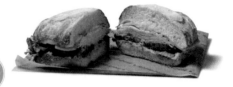

✔ Jersey Mike's Turkey Breast & Provolone Reduced Carb Wrap

MAINTAIN

525 calories
33 g fiber

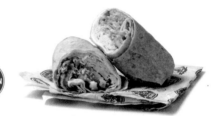

Other Good Choices

✓ 7-Eleven 7 Smart Turkey Sandwich **(300 calories, 2.5 g fat)**

✓ Sheetz Turkey Breast Sandwich on an herb sub roll with assorted fresh vegetables and yellow mustard **(300 calories)**

Sandwiches
GRILLED CHICKEN SANDWICHES AND WRAPS

❌ STOP EATING | ✅ START EATING

🏠 *Homemade*

❌ Panini made with 4 oz focaccia bread, 4 oz grilled chicken breast, 2 Tbsp pesto, and 2 oz provolone cheese (814 calories, 42 g fat)

✔ Panini made with 2 slices Arnold Stone Ground 100% Whole Wheat Bread, 3 oz grilled chicken breast, 1 Tbsp Tribe Sweet Roasted Red Pepper Hummus, 1 oz provolone cheese, lettuce, and tomato

STEADY LOSS

402 calories
14 g fat

✖ STOP EATING | ✔ START EATING

✖ Olive Garden Grilled Chicken Flatbread (760 calories, 51 g fat)

✖ Burger King TENDERCRISP Chicken Sandwich with mayo (660 calories, 40 g fat)

✖ Wendy's Grilled Asiago Ranch Chicken Club (540 calories, 22 g fat)

✔ Burger King TENDERGRILL Chicken Sandwich (order without mayo)

STEADY LOSS

350 calories
9 g fat

✔ Subway 6-inch Sweet Onion Chicken Teriyaki Sandwich

STEADY LOSS

370 calories
4.5 g fat

✔ ½ Applebee's Artisan Grilled Chicken Ciabatta

MAINTAIN

480 calories

Other Good Choices

✓ Panera Mediterranean Chicken Flatbread (**310 calories, 550 mg sodium**)

✓ Hardee's Charbroiled BBQ Chicken Sandwich (**320 calories, 4 g fat**)

✓ Wendy's Spicy Chicken Go Wrap (**340 calories, 16 g fat**)

✓ McDonald's Grilled Sweet Chili Chicken Premium McWrap (**400 calories**)

CHICKEN AND TUNA SALAD SANDWICHES

❌ STOP EATING | ✅ START EATING

🏠 *Homemade*

❌ Deli tuna salad on a whole wheat bagel, with lettuce and tomato (530 calories, 21 g fat)

✔ 2½ oz light tuna in water mixed with 1 Tbsp light mayonnaise on 2 slices Pepperidge Farm Very Thin 100% Whole Wheat with lettuce and tomato

KICK START

186 calories
3 g fat

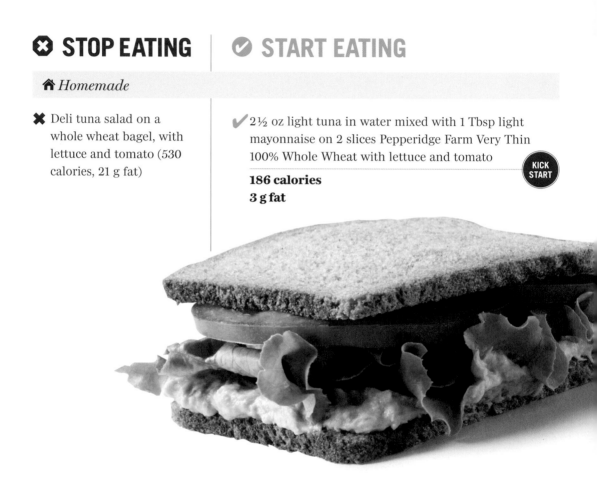

🛒 *Packaged*

✔ StarKist Ready-to-Eat Albacore Tuna Salad on ½ whole wheat bagel with lettuce and tomato

KICK START

245 calories
4.5 g fat

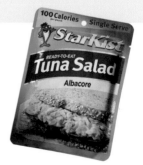

❌ STOP EATING | ✅ START EATING

❌ Boston Market All-White Chicken Salad Sandwich (890 calories, 56 g fat)

❌ Wawa Tuna on wheat with American cheese, lettuce and tomato (690 calories, 46 g fat)

❌ Potbelly Sandwich Flats Chicken Salad Sandwich (501 calories, 28 g fat)

✅ ½ Au Bon Pain Classic Chicken Salad Sandwich with cranberries

KICK START

220 calories 6 g fat

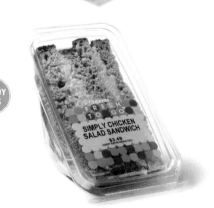

✅ 7-Eleven Chicken Salad Sandwich

STEADY LOSS

400 calories 14 g fat

Other Good Choices

✓ Choose Two portion McAlister's Tuna Salad Sandwich (**270 calories, 14 g fat**)

✓ Combo size Corner Bakery Café D.C. Chicken Salad on Steakhouse Rye Bread (**310 calories, 11 g fat**)

✓ Tim Horton Chicken Salad Sandwich (**340 calories, 9 g fat**)

Sandwiches
ROAST BEEF AND STEAK SANDWICHES

✖ STOP EATING | ### ✔ START EATING

✖ Roast beef sandwich made with kaiser roll, 3 oz fresh roast beef, 1 Tbsp mayo, lettuce, and tomato (465 calories, 21 g fat)

✔ Roast beef sandwich made with 2 slices Arnold Stone Ground 100% Whole Wheat Bread, 3 oz shaved deli roast beef, mustard, roasted peppers, lettuce, and tomato

256 calories
6 g fat

KICK START

❌ STOP EATING | ✅ START EATING

🛒 *Packaged*

❌ Stouffer's Philly-style Steak & Cheese Toasted Sub (370 calories)

✅ 1 (½ package) Lean Pockets Philly Steak & Cheese

STEADY LOSS

280 calories
8 g fat

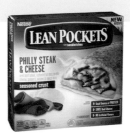

Other Good Choices

✓ Jimmy Dean BBQ Beef Sandwich (**300 calories**)

✓ Lean Cuisine Culinary Collection Philly-Style Steak & Cheese Panini (**320 calories**)

✓ Hot Pockets Philly Steak & Cheese in a Croissant Crust (**320 calories**)

🍴 *Restaurant*

❌ TGI Friday's French Dip Sandwich (740 calories, 1490 mg sodium)

❌ Subway 6-inch Philly Cheesesteak on 9-grain wheat bread with veggies (500 calories)

❌ Choose Two portion McAlister's Black Angus Club (400 calories, 20 g fat)

✅ Subway Kids Meal Roast Beef on 9-grain wheat bread with fresh veggies

KICK START

200 calories
3 g fat

✅ Arby's Roast Beef Classic Sandwich

MAINTAIN

360 calories

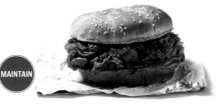

Other Good Choices

✓ Half size Au Bon Pain Black Angus Roast Beef and Herb Cheese sandwich (**260 calories, 7 g fat**)

✓ Hardee's Regular Roast Beef Sandwich (**300 calories, 14 g fat**)

✓ Subway 6-inch Roast Beef on 9-grain wheat bread with fresh veggies (**320 calories, 5 g fat**)

Sandwiches
HAM SANDWICHES

❌ STOP EATING	✅ START EATING

🛒 *Packaged*

❌ Lunchables Uploaded Lunch Combinations, 6-inch Ham + American Sub Sandwich (450 calories, 650 mg sodium)

✔ 1 (¼ package) Jimmy Dean Ham & Cheese Croissant Sandwich

KICK START

260 calories
610 mg sodium

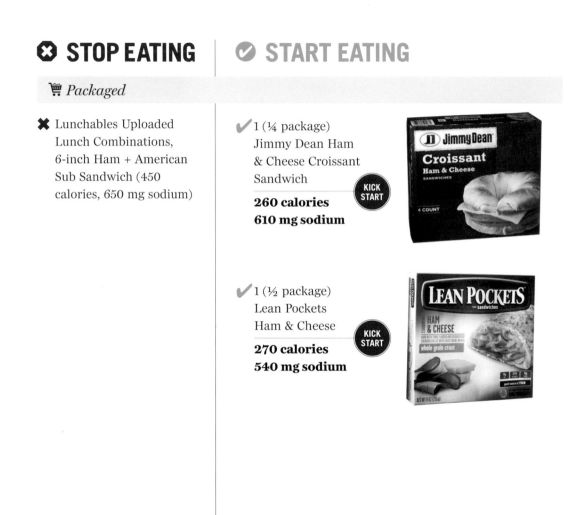

✔ 1 (½ package) Lean Pockets Ham & Cheese

KICK START

270 calories
540 mg sodium

✖ STOP EATING | ✔ START EATING

✗ *Restaurant*

✖ Wawa Classic Ham and Swiss, extra Swiss, mayo, and lettuce (1080 calories, 2379 mg sodium)

✖ Large (11 oz) supermarket deli ham and Swiss on a wheat roll (670 calories, 2370 mg sodium)

✖ Corner Bakery Café Mom's Smoked Ham on White Bread with mayo and Swiss cheese (580 calories, 2635 mg sodium)

✔ Subway 6-inch Black Forest Ham on 9-grain wheat bread with veggies **KICK START**

290 calories
800 mg sodium

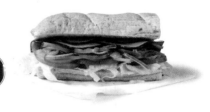

✔ Hardee's Hot Ham 'N' Cheese Sandwich **KICK START**

290 calories
1150 mg sodium

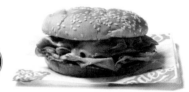

✔ Starbucks Ham and Swiss Panini **STEADY LOSS**

340 calories
1130 mg sodium

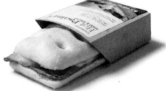

Other Good Choices

✓ Wawa Junior Ham and Swiss Sandwich on a wheat junior roll with honey mustard, veggies **(330 calories, 850 mg sodium)**

✓ Einstein Grab and Go Deli Ham Sandwich **(360 calories, 1190 mg sodium)**

Sandwiches
BLT SANDWICHES

❌ **STOP EATING**	✅ **START EATING**

❌ BLT made with 4 slices bacon, lettuce, and tomato, on 2 slices Pepperidge Farm Farmhouse Hearty White Bread with 2 Tbsp mayo (726 calories, 49 g fat)

✔ BLT made with 3 slices turkey bacon, lettuce, and tomato, on 2 slices Arnold Stone Ground 100% Whole Wheat Bread with 2 Tbsp mashed avocado

STEADY LOSS

240 calories
6.5 g fat

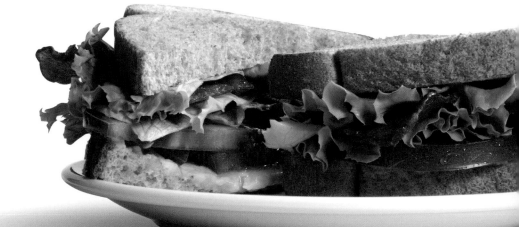

Choose Your Bacon

Not all bacon is created equal. See how many calories are in each slice of these common types of bacon.

Bacon	54
Canadian bacon	43
Vegetarian bacon	28
Turkey bacon	20

❌ STOP EATING | ✅ START EATING

❌ Applebee's American BLT (1080 calories, 74 g fat)

❌ Wawa Classic BLT on wheat classic roll with mayo, lettuce, and tomato (960 calories, 53 g fat)

❌ Five Guys BLT (533 calories, 34 g fat)

✔ Half size Panera Roasted Turkey & Avocado BLT on sourdough **KICK START**

250 calories
9 g fat

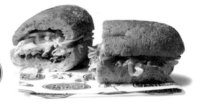

✔ Jersey Mike's Wheat Mini #1 BLT, no mayo **MAINTAIN**

440 calories

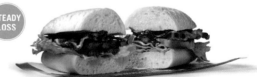

✔ Tim Horton BLT **STEADY LOSS**

360 calories
860 mg sodium

Other Good Choices

✓ McAlister's Choose Two portion BLT **(260 calories, 700 mg sodium)**

✓ Wawa Junior BLT on a wheat roll with spicy mustard, no cheese **(310 calories, 780 mg sodium)**

GRILLED CHEESE AND VEGGIE SANDWICHES

❌ STOP EATING | ✅ START EATING

🏠 *Homemade*

❌ Grilled cheese sandwich made with 2 slices Pepperidge Farm Farmhouse Hearty White Bread, 2 1-oz slices American cheese, and 2 Tbsp butter (631 calories, 40.5 g fat)

✔ Baked open-face sandwich made with 1 slice Pepperidge Farm Whole Grain Honey Wheat Bread, 3 Tbsp Kraft Shredded Reduced Fat Mild Cheddar, tomato slices, and roasted red peppers

KICK START

290 calories
10.5 g fat

Choose Your Cheese

Stop to consider what type of cheese you'd like on your sandwiches. See how many calories are in a 1-oz slice of your favorite cheese.

Cheddar 114	Muenster 104	Mozzarella 85
Swiss 108	Provolone 99	Reduced-fat Swiss 81
Jack 106	American 94	Reduced-fat provolone 78

✖ STOP EATING | ✔ START EATING

✗ *Restaurant*

✖ Starbucks Old-Fashioned
Grilled Cheese Sandwich
(580 calories, 29 g fat)

✖ Five Guys Cheese Veggie
Sandwich (510 calories,
21 g fat)

✔ Subway 6-inch
Veggie Delite on
9-grain wheat
bread

KICK START

**230 calories
2.5 g fat**

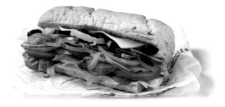

✔ Potbelly Flats
Mediterranean

MAINTAIN

**383 calories
13 g fat**

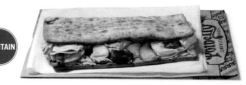

✔ Starbucks Roasted
Tomato &
Mozzarella
Panini

MAINTAIN

**390 calories
18 g fat**

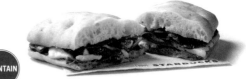

Other Good Choices

✓ Denny's Whole Wheat Bun with Cheddar Cheese (custom order)
(270 calories, 7 g fat)

✓ Half size Panera Mediterranean Veggie on Tomato Basil
(280 calories, 6 g fat)

✓ ½ Jersey Mike's Regular Veggie Sub on Wheat (order one, eat half)
(342 calories, 14.5 g fat)

Sandwiches
SLOPPY JOES

❌ STOP EATING | ### ✅ START EATING

🛒 *Packaged*

❌ ⅛ jar Stonewall Kitchen Sloppy Joe Sauce plus ⅓ pound 90% lean ground beef on a kaiser roll (402 calories)

❌ ¼ pouch NEAT Original Mix plus ¼ can tomato paste on a whole wheat hamburger bun (339 calories)

✔ 3 Tbsp Fantastic World Foods Vegetarian Sloppy Joe Mix, prepared, on a whole wheathamburger bun

194 calories

KICK START

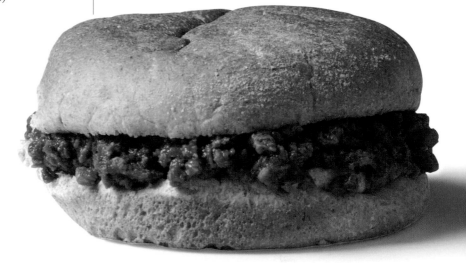

✅ START EATING

✅ 2¼ oz Hunt's Manwich Original Sloppy Joe Sauce plus 2¼ oz ground turkey breast on a whole wheat hamburger bun

218 calories

✅ 1 tsp McCormick Sweet & Smoky Sloppy Joes Skillet Sauce plus 3¼ oz 90% lean ground beef on a whole wheat hamburger bun

297 calories

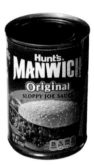

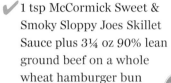

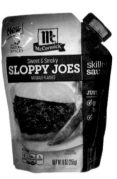

Other Good Choices

✅ ¼ container Hunt's Manwich Heat 'N Serve Original Sloppy Joe Sauce with Fully Cooked Ground Beef on a whole wheat hamburger bun **(257 calories)**

✅ 2¼ oz Hunt's Manwich Thick & Chunky Sloppy Joe Sauce plus 2¼ oz 90% lean ground beef on a whole wheat hamburger bun **(259 calories)**

✅ 2¼ oz Hunt's Manwich Bold Sloppy Joe Sauce plus 2¼ oz 80% lean ground beef on a whole wheat hamburger bun **(289 calories)**

Sandwiches
BURGERS

❌ STOP EATING | ✅ START EATING

🏠 *Homemade*

❌ Burger made with 4 oz 80% lean ground beef patty on a regular hamburger bun, topped with 2 slices American cheese, 2 Tbsp ketchup, lettuce, and tomato (571 calories)

✔ Burger made with 4 oz 95% lean ground beef patty on a whole wheat hamburger bun, topped with 1 Tbsp ketchup, ½ cup mushrooms (sautéed in ½ tsp olive oil), lettuce, and tomato

239 calories

(MAINTAIN)

Choose Your Meat

See how many calories are in one ounce of different types of cooked ground meat.

Ground pork.............................84	90% lean ground beef...............44	Ground turkey breast..................32
80% lean ground beef...............52	93% lean ground turkey............42	

❌ STOP EATING | ✅ START EATING

🛒 *Packaged*

❌ BUBBA Original Burger patty, no bun (420 calories)

✅ Boca All American Flame Grilled Veggie Burger patty, no bun

120 calories
5 g fat

MAINTAIN

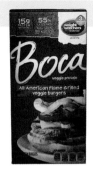

Other Good Choices

✓ MorningStar Farms Grillers Original patty, no bun **(130 calories)**

✓ Amy's All American Veggie Burger patty, no bun **(140 calories)**

✓ BUBBA Turkey Burger patty, no bun **(190 calories)**

🍴 *Restaurant*

❌ TGI Friday's Sedona Black Bean Burger (1260 calories, 3320 mg sodium)

❌ Five Guys Hamburger (700 calories)

❌ Burger King Whopper, with mayo (650 calories)

✅ White Castle Double Original Slider

240 calories

KICK START

✅ Burger King Whopper Jr., with mayo

300 calories

STEADY LOSS

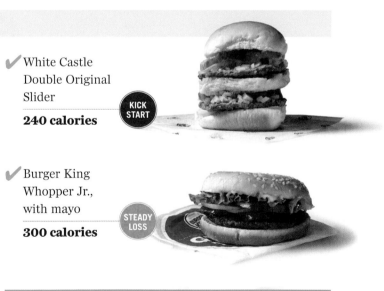

Other Good Choices

✓ Wendy's Jr. Cheeseburger **(280 calories)**

✓ McDonald's Cheeseburger **(290 calories)**

✓ Burger King Double Hamburger **(320 calories)**

✓ In-N-Out Hamburger w/Onion **(390 calories)**

❌ STOP EATING | ✅ START EATING

🛒 *Packaged*

❌ 1 Ballpark Beef Frank, no bun (190 calories, 16 g fat)

❌ 1 Nathan's Natural Casing Beef Frankfurters, no bun (150 calories)

✅ 1 Applegate Natural Uncured Beef Hot Dog, no bun

KICK START

70 calories

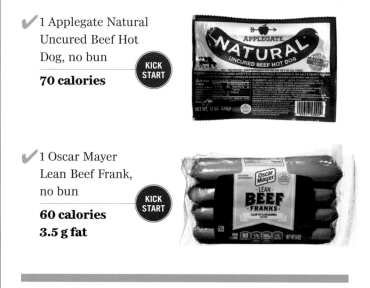

✅ 1 Oscar Mayer Lean Beef Frank, no bun

KICK START

60 calories
3.5 g fat

Other Good Choices

✓ 1 Oscar Mayer Bun Length Turkey Frank, no bun (**120 calories, 9 g fat**)

✓ 1 Hebrew National Reduced Fat Beef Frank, no bun (**110 calories, 9 g fat**)

✖ STOP EATING

✗ *Restaurant*

✖ Sonic Footlong Quarter Pound Coney with bun (830 calories, 55 g fat)

✖ Five Guys Hot Dog with bun (545 calories)

✖ Hardee's Jumbo Chili Dog with bun (370 calories)

✔ START EATING

✔ Five Guys Bunless Hot Dogs

STEADY LOSS

285 calories

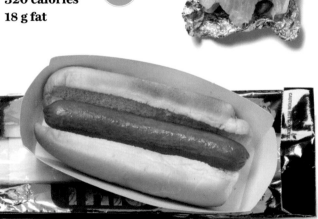

✔ Sonic All Beef Regular Hot Dog with bun

STEADY LOSS

320 calories

18 g fat

Chapter 12
MAIN DISHES

BBQ ribs. Fried chicken. Spaghetti and meatballs. Alfredo sauce. Pizza. There's almost no way that you're going to find healthy versions of these on restaurant menus. And portions can be so big that you'll get all your calories for the day, and more, if you eat the whole thing. So I know that if I want one of these, I have to limit how much I eat. That means really small portions or maybe just a taste of what's on my husband's plate. Then I pair it with a big salad and fruit for dessert to round out my meal nutritionally and fill me up.

If you eat restaurant food, you have to find ways to swap out the fat! Guess how restaurants make steak, chicken, and fish moist and juicy? With extra butter. That's why it's important to ask questions when you order so that you can avoid fat land mines. Every tablespoon of butter on your dish is another 100 calories, and that's a lot if you're trying to keep your meal to 400 or 500 calories. Also, avoid one-dish meals like pot pies and casseroles in restaurants because it's impossible to know exactly how the chef prepared them.

My go-to mains are chicken breast, fish, and pork tenderloin because in their natural state they're pretty low in fat and calories. Salmon is my favorite; it has great flavor and MUFAs. Sometimes I order white-flesh fish such as tilapia, cod, haddock, snapper, or flounder because they are so low in fat and calories that I can eat a larger portion. Of course I have to swap for a smaller portion if I can't avoid the butter or creamy sauce on top.

In Chinese restaurants, I eat fist-size portions of rice and one main dish, and avoid dishes with the word *crispy* or *fried* in their name. When I order Mexican, I stick with a palm-size protein portion, one carb side (one tortilla or 1 cup beans or rice, but not both), lots of veggies, and a bit of guacamole.

Also, I've found that side dishes are often calorie-laden and portions are out of control. Pay careful attention in this chapter to the portions I list. And note that the default listing is the entrée only, with no sides. (In a few cases, we made exceptions.) That gives you some room to order healthier side dishes, such as steamed veggies or a side salad.

Two rules to follow when you cook meat, poultry, and fish at home: Choose lean cuts or parts, and minimize extra fat added during cooking. A set of nonstick pans and a generous spritz of cooking spray go a long way! Also, look for recipes that were developed for leaner cuts like London broil, skinless chicken, and white-flesh fish like tilapia and sole because they may have tricks for keeping in the moisture. For instance, keep the skin on lean cuts of chicken and turkey while you cook, which helps keep the flesh nice and moist. Then remove the skin before eating.

When comparing frozen dinners and other packaged main dishes, consider the proportion of the main entrée to the sides and opt for those with the simplest sounding veggies. You may need to add a side salad or other vegetable to round out these meals nutritionally, though.

STOP EATING	START EATING
• Oversized protein portions, especially of hopelessly high-fat foods like ribs and marbled steak	• Protein portions the size of a deck of cards
• Higher-fat types of ground meat, such as pork and chuck, in meatloaf, meatballs, and sauce	• Ground beef that is at least 90% lean, or ground poultry
• Fried or roast chicken or turkey with the skin on	• Roast chicken or turkey with the skin on during cooking but off before eating
• Fish basted with butter or oil, or fried	• Plain grilled, broiled, or steamed fish, garnished with fresh herbs or low-fat sauces
• Thick-crust pizza with extra cheese: Remember that every ounce of crust equals a slice of bread, and a generous slice could have 4 ounces of crust!	• A thin slice of thin-crust pizza with vegetables (and ask for less cheese, if possible)
• A big bowl of any type of pasta, particularly when topped with a cream or meat sauce	• A fist-size pasta portion with tomato sauce
• Chinese or Mexican meals with big portions and lots of different dishes	• Modest portions of Chinese or Mexican foods, and limits on high-carb and fried dishes such as egg rolls, fried rice, noodle dishes, chimichangas, and chips
• Main-dish-only meals of protein and starch like spaghetti and meatballs or fettuccine Alfredo, with no veggie side dishes	• Small main-dish portions paired with a filling salad or vegetable side dish

Main Dishes
STEAK

❌ STOP EATING | ✅ START EATING

🛒 *Packaged*

❌ Stouffer's Satisfying Servings Bourbon Steak Tips with mashed potatoes (490 calories, 890 mg sodium)

❌ Evol Fire Grilled Steak with black beans and red peppers (400 calories, 20 g fat)

❌ Marie Callender's frozen Steak & Roasted Potatoes with green beans (350 calories)

✅ Banquet Salisbury Steak Meal with mashed potatoes and corn

STEADY LOSS

230 calories
9 g fat

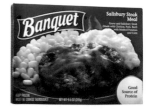

✅ Healthy Choice Café Steamers Barbecue Seasoned Steak with red potatoes

KICK START

260 calories
3.5 g fat

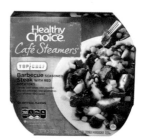

Other Good Choices

✓ Lean Cuisine Comfort Steak Portabello **(160 calories, 610 mg sodium)**

✓ Weight Watchers Smart Ones Salisbury Steak **(250 calories)**

✓ Lean Cuisine Culinary Collection Salisbury Steak with Macaroni & Cheese **(260 calories)**

❌ STOP EATING | ✅ START EATING

🍴 *Restaurant*

❌ Macaroni Grill Calabrese Steak with potatoes and vegetables (1650 calories, 1820 mg sodium)

❌ LongHorn Steakhouse 11 oz Ribeye Steak (740 calories, 49 g fat)

❌ 8 oz Outback Steakhouse Herb-Roasted Prime Rib, no sides (704 calories, 57 g fat)

✔ Panda Express kids' meal Shanghai Angus Steak

STEADY LOSS

240 calories

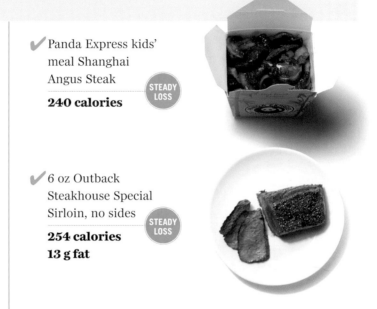

✔ 6 oz Outback Steakhouse Special Sirloin, no sides

STEADY LOSS

254 calories
13 g fat

Other Good Choices

✓ Chili's Lighter Choice 6 oz Classic Sirloin, with side dishes **(240 calories, 7 g fat)**

✓ Applebee's 7 oz House Sirloin **(280 calories, 15 g fat)**

✓ Pei Wei Ginger Broccoli with steak and rice (order one small, eat half) **(335 calories)**

Choose Your Cut

See how many calories are in each cut of steak, per 3 ounces cooked.

Porterhouse	180	London broil	157
Ribeye	165	Top sirloin	156
Filet mignon	164	Sirloin tip	150
Tri-tip	158		

Main Dishes
MEATLOAF

❌ STOP EATING | ✅ START EATING

🏠 Homemade

❌ 1 serving (1/10 recipe) meatloaf made with 1 lb each ground pork and 80% lean ground beef and 1 packet McCormick Meat Loaf Seasoning Mix (184 calories)

✔ 1 serving (1/10 recipe) meatloaf made with 93% lean ground turkey and McCormick Meat Loaf Seasoning Mix

KICK START

130 calories

Choose Your Meat

Make sure your meat is no mystery. See how many calories per ounce are in common cooked ground meats.

Ground pork	84
80% lean ground beef	52
90% lean ground beef	44
93% lean ground turkey	42
Ground turkey breast	32

HOW TO MAKE IT

Combine 2 pounds 93% lean ground turkey with 1 packet McCormick Meat Loaf Seasoning Mix. Place in a loaf pan and bake in a 350°F oven until the internal temperature reaches at least 140°F, about 1 hour. (Makes 10 servings)

❌ STOP EATING | ✓ START EATING

🛒 *Packaged*

❌ Stouffer's Satisfying Servings Meatloaf with mashed potatoes (540 calories, 26 g fat)

❌ Marie Callender's frozen Meat Loaf and Gravy with mashed potatoes and veggies (450 calories)

❌ Amy's Veggie Loaf with mashed potatoes, corn, and peas (340 calories)

✓ Lean Cuisine Comfort Meatloaf with Mashed Potatoes

240 calories
7 g fat

STEADY LOSS

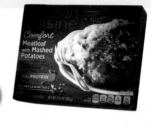

✓ Hormel Compleats Meatloaf & Gravy with Mashed Potatoes

280 calories
12 g fat

MAINTAIN

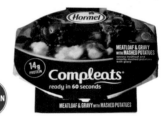

Other Good Choices

✓ Weight Watchers Smart Ones Meatloaf (**270 calories, 9 g fat**)

✓ Banquet Meat Loaf Meal (**280 calories, 13 g fat**)

🍴 *Restaurant*

❌ Large Boston Market Meatloaf with potato and corn (760 calories)

✓ Regular Boston Market Meatloaf with potato and corn

510 calories

MAINTAIN

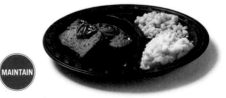

Other Good Choice

✓ Bob Evans Meatloaf & Gravy (**500 calories**)

Main Dishes
PORK CHOPS AND BARBECUE RIBS

❌ STOP EATING	✅ START EATING

🛒 *Packaged*

STOP EATING

✖ Banquet Double Meat Pork Rib Meal, with sides (480 calories, 23 g fat)

✖ Marie Callender's frozen Country Fried Pork Chop & Gravy with mashed potatoes and cinnamon glazed apples (460 calories, 12 g sugars)

START EATING

✔ 3 oz portion (about ⅒ package) Tyson Pork Roast Kit with vegetables

STEADY LOSS

300 calories
0 g sugars

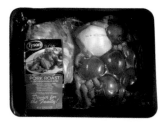

✔ Banquet Boneless Pork Riblet Meal, with sides

STEADY LOSS

310 calories
11 g fat

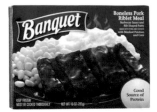

✖ STOP EATING ┃ ✔ START EATING

✗ *Restaurant*

✖ TGI Friday's Jack Daniel's Ribs (1590 calories, 3080 mg sodium)

✖ Macaroni Grill Chianti Pork Chop (960 calories)

✖ Ruby Tuesday Hickory Bourbon-Glazed Pork Chop, with mashed potatoes and green beans (885 calories, 42 g fat)

✔ Longhorn Steakhouse Cowboy Pork Chops, no sides

MAINTAIN

400 calories
14 g fat

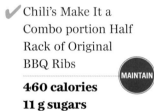

✔ Chili's Make It a Combo portion Half Rack of Original BBQ Ribs

MAINTAIN

460 calories
11 g sugars

Other Good Choices

✓ Hometown Buffet Carved Grilled Pork Loin **(140 calories)**

✓ Texas Roadhouse Grilled Pork Chops **(450 calories)**

Main Dishes
FISH AND SHELLFISH

⊗ STOP EATING | ✓ START EATING

🏠 Homemade

✖ 1 serving (¼ recipe) linguine with clam sauce, made with garlic and anchovies sautéed in ¼ cup olive oil, plus 1 cup each white wine and clam juice, 1 15-oz can baby clams, and 1 pound linguine (710 calories)

✓ ½ cup (about ⅓ can) Cento White Clam Sauce on 1 cup cooked linguine **MAINTAIN**

381 calories

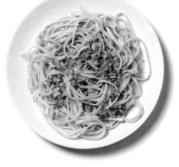

🛒 Packaged

✖ Marie Callender's frozen Golden Battered Fish Fillets, with broccoli, cheese sauce, and rice (410 calories, 1260 mg sodium)

✖ Stouffer's Classic Fish Filet with macaroni and cheese (400 calories, 19 g fat)

✖ ½ package Bertolli Shrimp Scampi & Linguine (480 calories)

✓ 1 Blue Horizon Maryland Style Crab Cake **KICK START**

160 calories

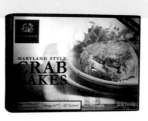

✓ Lean Cuisine Marketplace Parmesan Crusted Fish **STEADY LOSS**

290 calories
570 mg sodium

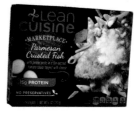

Other Good Choices

✓ Michelina's Lean Gourmet Shrimp with Pasta and Vegetables **(240 calories)**

✓ 1 SeaPak Maryland Style Crab Cake + ½ package sauce **(240 calories)**

✓ Healthy Choice Herb Crusted Fish **(270 calories, 370 mg sodium)**

✓ Atkins Shrimp Scampi **(310 calories)**

❌ STOP EATING | ✅ START EATING

✗ *Restaurant*

❌ Joe's Crab Shack Cedar Roasted Salmon (1500 calories, 119 g fat)

❌ Macaroni Grill Mediterranean Branzino (900 calories)

❌ Bonefish Grill Spicy Tuna Bowl (841 calories, 24 g fat)

❌ Joe's Crab Shack Popcorn Shrimp (1340 calories, 4750 mg sodium)

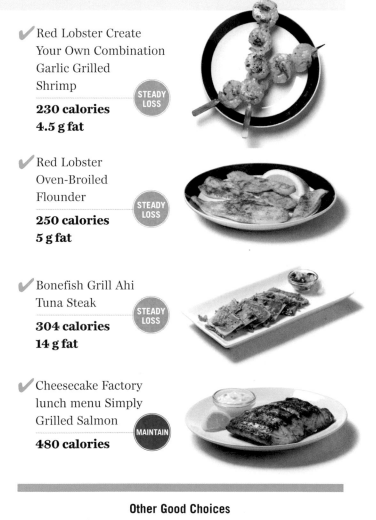

✔ Red Lobster Create Your Own Combination Garlic Grilled Shrimp **STEADY LOSS**

230 calories
4.5 g fat

✔ Red Lobster Oven-Broiled Flounder **STEADY LOSS**

250 calories
5 g fat

✔ Bonefish Grill Ahi Tuna Steak **STEADY LOSS**

304 calories
14 g fat

✔ Cheesecake Factory lunch menu Simply Grilled Salmon **MAINTAIN**

480 calories

Other Good Choices

✓ Red Lobster Create Your Own Combination Portion Wood-Grilled Fresh Salmon **(310 calories)**

✓ Bonefish Grill Chilean Sea Bass **(345 calories)**

✓ Chili's Lighter Choice Salmon **(340 calories, 19 g fat)**

Main Dishes
CHICKEN AND TURKEY

❌ STOP EATING | ✅ START EATING

🛒 *Packaged*

❌ Hungry Man Selects Classic Fried Chicken (840 calories, 41 g fat)

❌ Marie Callender's frozen Country Fried Chicken & Gravy, with corn (570 calories, 7 g sugars)

❌ Marie Callender's frozen Roasted Turkey Breast & Stuffing, with gravy, potatoes, and veggies (320 calories)

❌ Lean Cuisine Marketplace Orange Chicken (310 calories)

Choose Your Pieces

A lot of the fat in chicken and turkey comes from the skin. See how many calories are in different pieces of roasted chicken or turkey.

Turkey thigh, skinless	526
Chicken thigh, with skin	313
Turkey drumstick, skinless	286
Chicken thigh, skinless	208
Chicken drumstick, with skin	201
Chicken breast, with skin	193
Chicken drumstick, skinless	150
Chicken breast, skinless	142
Turkey wing, skinless	88

✔ Weight Watchers Smart Ones Slow Roasted Turkey Breast

KICK START

210 calories

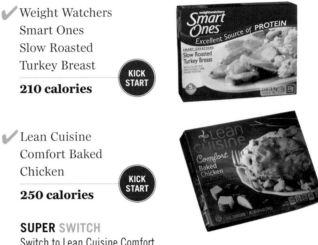

✔ Lean Cuisine Comfort Baked Chicken

KICK START

250 calories

SUPER SWITCH
Switch to Lean Cuisine Comfort Herb Roasted Chicken and drop another 80 calories!

✔ Stouffer's Classic Fried Chicken Breast, with potato and gravy

STEADY LOSS

350 calories
1 g sugars

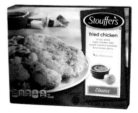

Other Good Choices

✓ Hormel Compleats Chicken Breast & Mashed Potatoes **(210 calories)**

✓ Banquet Turkey Meal, with potatoes and peas **(230 calories)**

✓ Stouffer's Classic Baked Chicken Breast with gravy and mashed potatoes **(240 calories)**

✓ Healthy Choice Country Fried Chicken **(340 calories, 8 g fat)**

❌ STOP EATING | ✓ START EATING

✗ *Restaurant*

❌ Chili's Honey-Chipotle Chicken Crispers, with corn, fries, and dipping sauce (1560 calories, 4960 mg sodium)

❌ IHOP Fried Chicken Dinner (1500 calories, 85 g fat)

❌ TGI Friday's Sizzling Chicken and Shrimp (1140 calories, 77 g fat)

❌ Maggiano's Lighter Take Chicken Piccata (580 calories, 23 g fat)

❌ Boston Market 3 piece (2 thighs, 1 drumstick) Dark Rotisserie Chicken (540 calories, 36 g fat)

Other Good Choices

✓ Carrabba's small Wood-Grilled Chicken (**179 calories, 4 g fat**)

✓ Chili's Lighter Choice Margarita Grilled Chicken, no sides (**190 calories**)

✓ Bob Evans Fried Chicken Breast (**230 calories**)

✓ KFC Original Recipe Chicken Breast

MAINTAIN

320 calories

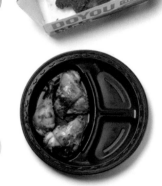

✓ Boston Market 3 piece (2 thighs, 1 drumstick) Dark Rotisserie Chicken (remove skin before eating)

STEADY LOSS

340 calories
17 g fat

SUPER SWITCH
Switch to Boston Market Quarter White Rotisserie Chicken (Skinless) and drop another 120 calories

✓ Chick-fil-A Chick-n-Strips with 1 packet Barbeque Sauce

MAINTAIN

405 calories

✓ TGI Friday's Sizzling Chicken and Spinach

KICK START

410 calories
15 g fat

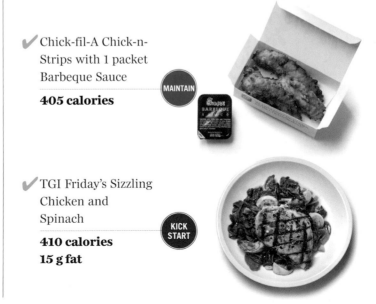

Main Dishes
POT PIES, CASSEROLES, AND TETRAZZINI

✖ STOP EATING	✔ START EATING

🛒 *Packaged*

✖ Stouffer's Satisfying Servings White Meat Chicken Pot Pie (590 calories, 34 g fat)

✖ Stouffer's Classics Tuna Noodle Casserole (450 calories)

✖ Amy's Vegetable Pot Pie (430 calories, 20 g fat)

✔ Weight Watchers Smart Ones Tuna Noodle Casserole

250 calories

(STEADY LOSS)

✔ 1 cup (⅕ box) prepared Tuna Helper Tetrazzini

280 calories
2 g fat

(STEADY LOSS)

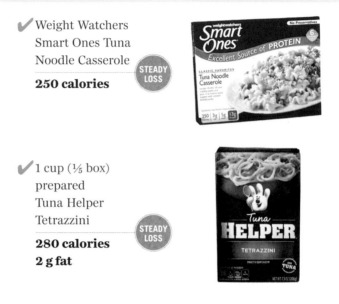

✅ START EATING

🛒 *Packaged*

✔ Healthy Choice Café
Steamers Crustless
Chicken Pot Pie

280 calories
7 g fiber

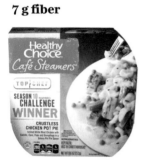

✔ Stouffer's Classics
Turkey Tetrazzini

390 calories

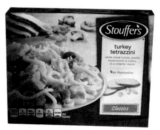

Other Good Choices

✓ Weight Watchers Smart Ones Crustless Chicken Pot Pie
(200 calories)

✓ Atkins Crustless Chicken Pot Pie **(330 calories)**

Main Dishes
CHICKEN AND EGGPLANT PARMIGIANA

❌ **STOP EATING**	✅ **START EATING**

🛒 *Packaged*

✖ ½ package Newman's Own Chicken Parmigiana & Penne Complete Skillet Meal (490 calories, 25 g fat)

✔ CedarLane Eggplant Parmesan

KICK START

280 calories
13 g fat

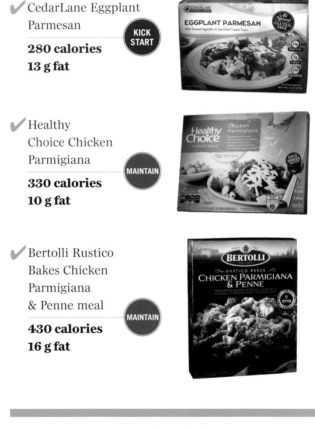

✔ Healthy Choice Chicken Parmigiana

MAINTAIN

330 calories
10 g fat

✔ Bertolli Rustico Bakes Chicken Parmigiana & Penne meal

MAINTAIN

430 calories
16 g fat

Other Good Choices

✓ Artisan Bistro Chicken Parmesan Bake (**200 calories, 6 g fat**)

✓ Weight Watchers Smart Ones Chicken Parmesan (**280 calories, 5 g fat**)

⊗ STOP EATING | ⊘ START EATING

✗ *Restaurant*

✗ Macaroni Grill Eggplant
Parmesan (1340 calories,
1520 mg sodium)

✔ Olive Garden lunch menu Eggplant Parmigiana
(order one, eat half)

395 calories

STEADY
LOSS

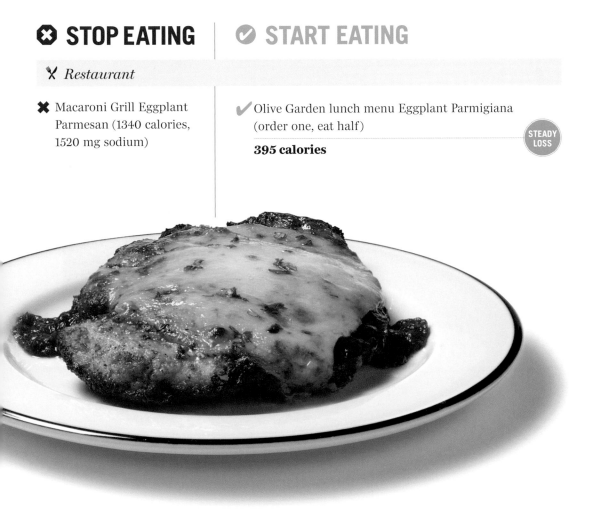

Other Good Choice

✓ Carrabba's lunch menu Chicken Parmesan, no pasta
(321 calories, 15 mg sodium)

Main Dishes
PIZZA

⊗ STOP EATING	⊘ START EATING

🛒 *Packaged*

STOP EATING

✖ Weight Watchers Smart Ones Pepperoni Pizza (430 calories)

✖ ⅓ Freschetta Thin & Crispy 4 Cheese Medley Pizza (370 calories)

START EATING

✔ ⅓ Kashi Thin Crust Pizza Margherita **KICK START**

260 calories
4 g fiber

✔ ⅓ Newman's Own Thin & Crispy Uncured Pepperoni Pizza **MAINTAIN**

320 calories

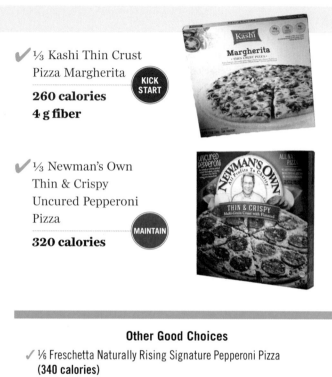

Other Good Choices

✓ ⅙ Freschetta Naturally Rising Signature Pepperoni Pizza **(340 calories)**

✓ Lean Cuisine Simple Favorites French Bread Cheese Pizza **(340 calories)**

✓ ¼ Red Baron Classic Crust Pepperoni Pizza **(370 calories)**

Choose Your Toppings

Toppings can double or triple the calories of a pizza, depending on what you choose. See how many calories common toppings have per ounce.

Pepperoni	144	Ham	45
Bacon	135	Roasted red peppers	7
Shredded cheese	110	Green peppers	7
Olives	50	Mushrooms	5

✖ STOP EATING | ✔ START EATING

🍴 *Restaurant*

✖ Pizza Hut Veggie Lover's
6-inch Personal Pan
Pizza (550 calories)

✖ ¼ thin crust
California Pizza Kitchen
Meat Cravers pizza
(399 calories)

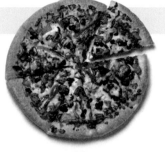

✔ ⅛ of medium
12-inch pan Pizza
Hut Veggie
Lover's pizza

KICK START

230 calories

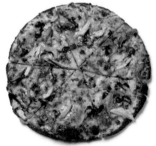

✔ ¼ thin crust
California Pizza
Kitchen Roasted
Artichoke + Spinach
with Chicken

STEADY LOSS

302 calories

SUPER SWITCH
Switch to ¼ regular California Pizza Kitchen Wild Mushroom Pizza and
drop another 46 calories

Other Good Choices

✓ ¼ of small Domino's Build-Your-Own Pizza with crunchy thin
crust, marinara sauce, regular cheese, spinach and mushrooms
(206 calories)

✓ ⅛ of medium 12-inch Thin 'N Crispy Pizza Hut Veggie Lover's pizza
(180 calories)

Main Dishes
PASTA

❌ **STOP EATING** | ✅ **START EATING**

🏠 *Homemade*

❌ 1 cup cooked spaghetti with ⅔ cup each ground pork and marinara sauce (749 calories, 17 g sugars)

✓ ½ cup each cooked Barilla Protein PLUS spaghetti, 93% lean ground turkey, and Barilla Traditional Sauce

348 calories
8 g sugars

STEADY LOSS

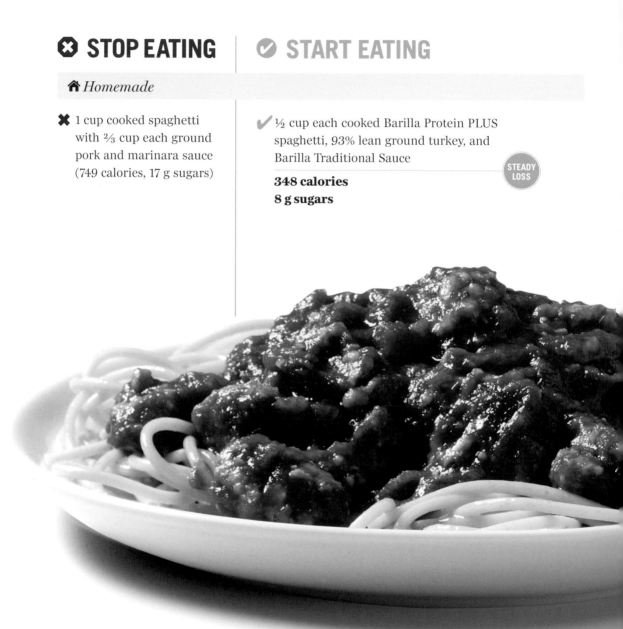

✖ STOP EATING | ✔ START EATING

🛒 Packaged

✖ Stouffer's Satisfying Servings Chicken Fettuccine Alfredo (650 calories, 32 g fat)

✖ Marie Callender's frozen Spaghetti & Meatballs (420 calories, 13 g fat)

✔ Banquet Fettuccine Alfredo **STEADY LOSS**

290 calories
12 g fat

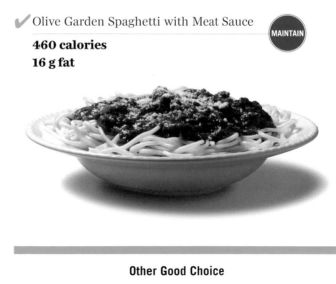

✔ Evol Butternut Squash and Sage Ravioli bowl **STEADY LOSS**

320 calories
9 g fat

Other Good Choices

✓ Hormel Compleats Spaghetti & Meat Sauce **(230 calories, 7 g fat)**

✓ Lean Cuisine Simple Favorites Cheese Ravioli **(250 calories, 6 g fat)**

✓ Amy's Vegetable Lasagna **(370 calories)**

🍴 Restaurant

✖ Maggiano's Taylor Street Baked Ziti (1410 calories, 4060 mg sodium)

✖ Bertucci's Four Cheese Ravioli (950 calories)

✖ Olive Garden lunch menu Spaghetti with Meatballs (740 calories, 35 g fat)

✔ Olive Garden Spaghetti with Meat Sauce **MAINTAIN**

460 calories
16 g fat

Other Good Choice

✓ Maggiano's Mushroom Ravioli al Forno **(375 calories)**

Main Dishes
MAC 'N' CHEESE

✖ STOP EATING | ✔ START EATING

🛒 *Packaged*

STOP EATING:

✖ Hormel Compleats Macaroni & Cheese (440 calories, 20 g fat)

✖ 1 cup prepared Kraft Macaroni & Cheese dinner (400 calories, 18 g fat)

START EATING:

✔ Kraft Macaroni & Cheese Original Dinner Cup **STEADY LOSS**
220 calories
4 g fat

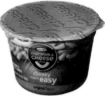

✔ 1 cup prepared Annie's Shells & Real Aged Cheddar, made with ¼ cup skim milk and 1½ tsp butter **STEADY LOSS**
270 calories
4.5 g fat

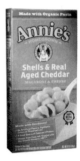

✔ 1 cup prepared Hodgson Mill Whole Wheat Macaroni & Cheese, made with ¼ cup skim milk and 1½ tsp butter **MAINTAIN**
325 calories
8 g fat

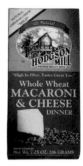

Other Good Choices

✔ 2¼ cups Green Giant Steamers Macaroni and Cheese Sauce with Broccoli (**250 calories, 5 g fat**)

✔ Weight Watchers Smart Ones Macaroni & Cheese (**260 calories, 2 g fat**)

✔ Banquet Macaroni & Cheese Meal (**260 calories, 6 g fat**)

❌ STOP EATING | ✓ START EATING

✖ Longhorn Steakhouse
Mac & Cheese
(610 calories, 37 g fat,
1210 mg sodium)

✖ Macaroni Grill Child's
Macaroni and Cheese
(540 calories, 1190 mg
sodium)

✖ Ruby Tuesday Baked
Mac 'n Cheese
(465 calories, 28 g fat)

✓ Corner Bakery Café Mac & Three Cheese

290 calories
400 mg sodium

STEADY
LOSS

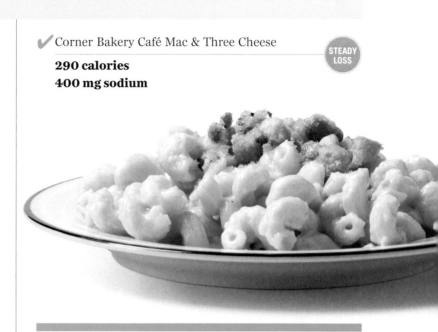

Other Good Choices

✓ Bob Evans Special Recipe Macaroni and Cheese **(280 calories, 15 g fat)**

✓ Boston Market Macaroni and Cheese **(280 calories, 11 g fat)**

✓ Olive Garden Kids' Macaroni & Cheese **(350 calories, 8 g fat)**

Main Dishes
MEXICAN FOOD

❌ STOP EATING	✅ START EATING

🛒 *Packaged*

STOP EATING

❌ ½ package Old El Paso Chicken Quesadillas (620 calories, 30 g fat)

❌ Evol Spicy Steak Big Burrito (610 calories)

❌ 1 Old El Paso Chicken Burrito (½ package) (480 calories, 1050 mg sodium)

START EATING

✔ Amy's Bean & Cheese Burrito

**310 calories
9 g fat**

STEADY LOSS

✔ ½ package Newman's Own Chicken Fajita Complete Skillet Meal

**310 calories
6 g fat**

STEADY LOSS

✔ Stouffer's Fit Kitchen Steak Fajita

370 calories

STEADY LOSS

Other Good Choices

✓ 1⅔ cups (⅙ package) Birds Eye Voila! Fajita Chicken **(170 calories, 2 g fat)**

✓ Tina's Bean & Cheese Burrito **(260 calories, 7 g fat)**

❌ STOP EATING | ✅ START EATING

❌ Applebee's Sizzling Skillet Steak Fajitas (1330 calories, 5240 mg sodium)

❌ 3 Chipotle Crispy Corn Tacos with carnitas, brown rice, black beans, fajita vegetables, sour cream (875 calories, 37.5 g fat)

❌ El Pollo Loco Spicy Chipotle Chicken Burrito (860 calories, 2500 mg sodium)

✅ ⅓ order Chili's Fresh Mex Fajitas with Grilled Steak, peppers, onions, and toppings and 1 tortilla **STEADY LOSS**

327 calories
21 g fat

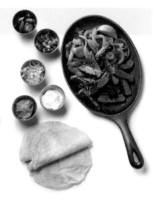

✅ Chipotle salad made with barbacoa, brown rice, fajita vegetables, fresh tomato salsa, lettuce **STEADY LOSS**

415 calories
14.5 g fat

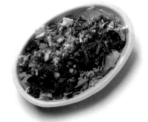

Other Good Choices

✓ 1 Chili's Chicken Soft Taco (Southwest Pairings menu) **(260 calories, 11 g fat)**

✓ On the Border Chicken Fajitas **(320 calories, 770 mg sodium)**

✓ On the Border Green Chile Carnitas Taco (ask for half the rice) **(385 calories)**

✓ El Pollo Loco Chicken Tostada Salad, no dressing or shell **(430 calories, 1130 mg sodium)**

Choose Your Tortilla

Think all tortillas have about the same number of calories? Think again. See how many calories are in different sizes and types of tortillas.

10-inch flour tortilla	217
7-inch flour tortilla	147
8-inch low-carb tortilla	130
6-inch flour tortilla	90
6-inch corn tortilla	52
4½-inch corn tortilla	44

Main Dishes
CHINESE FOOD

❌ STOP EATING | ✅ START EATING

🏠 Homemade

❌ Stir-fry made with ½ cup dark meat chicken with skin, 1 cup stir-fry vegetables, ½ cup sweet and sour sauce, 2 Tbsp oil for frying, and 1 cup white rice (810 calories, 48 g fat)

✔ Stir-fry made with ½ cup cubed firm tofu, 2 cups fresh or 1½ cups frozen assorted stir-fry vegetables, (no sauce or seasoning), 1 tsp oil for stir-frying, 1 Tbsp teriyaki sauce, and ½ cup brown rice

STEADY LOSS

235 calories
11 g fat

Choose Your Sauce

While the differences listed below may not seem like much, some sauces can add up to hundreds of calories in a whole dish. See how many calories are in different sauces per tablespoon.

Peanut sauce	46
Duck sauce	40
Hoisin sauce	35
Sweet and sour sauce	19
Teriyaki sauce	16
Szechuan sauce	15
Chili garlic sauce	15
Soy sauce	8

❌ STOP EATING | ✅ START EATING

🛒 *Packaged*

❌ ½ package Newman's Own General Paul's Chicken Complete Skillet Meal (400 calories, 16 g fat)

❌ Healthy Choice Sesame Chicken (410 calories, 10 g fat)

Other Good Choices

✓ Weight Watchers Smart Ones Chicken Oriental **(250 calories, 2.5 g fat)**

✓ Lean Cuisine Culinary Collection Chicken with Almonds **(290 calories)**

✅ ½ package Newman's Own Beef & Broccoli Complete Skillet Meal

KICK START

250 calories
100% vitamin C

✅ Healthy Choice Café Steamers General Tso's Spicy Chicken

STEADY LOSS

290 calories
3.5 g fat

🍴 *Restaurant*

❌ PF Chang's Crispy Honey Chicken (1140 calories)

❌ Panda Express Beijing Beef (470 calories, 26 g fat)

✅ ½ order PF Chang's Almond and Cashew Chicken

STEADY LOSS

320 calories

Other Good Choices

✓ Panda Express String Bean Chicken Breast **(190 calories)**

✓ Pei Wei Sweet & Sour Original with Vegetables & Tofu (order one, eat half) **(282 calories)**

Main Dishes
JAPANESE FOOD

⊗ STOP EATING	⊘ START EATING

🛒 *Packaged*

✖ ½ package Newman's Own Grilled Chicken Teriyaki with Lo Mein Noodles Complete Skillet Meal (360 calories, 20 g sugars)

✔ Healthy Choice Café Steamers Beef Teriyaki

270 calories
5 g fat

(STEADY LOSS)

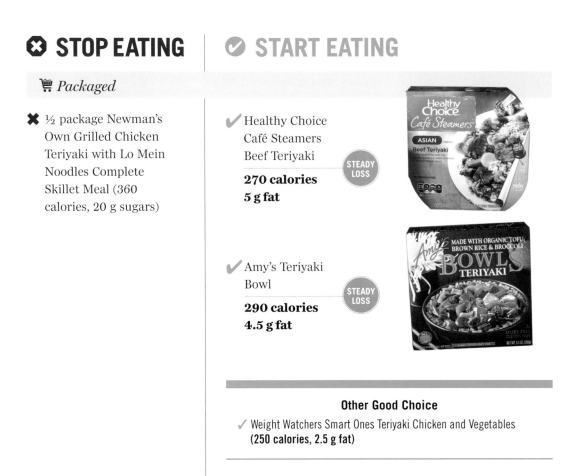

✔ Amy's Teriyaki Bowl

290 calories
4.5 g fat

(STEADY LOSS)

Other Good Choice

✓ Weight Watchers Smart Ones Teriyaki Chicken and Vegetables (250 calories, 2.5 g fat)

❌ STOP EATING | ✅ START EATING

🍴 *Restaurant*

❌ Benihana Chateaubriand (370 calories)

❌ 1 (6 pieces) Philadelphia (salmon and cream cheese) sushi roll (287 calories, 7 g fat)

❌ 1 (6 pieces) spicy tuna roll (254 calories)

✅ 4 pieces salmon sashimi

KICK START

108 calories

✅ 1 (6 pieces) tuna avocado roll

KICK START

173 calories
3.5 g fat

✅ Benihana Hibachi Steak, with mixed vegetables

KICK START

240 calories

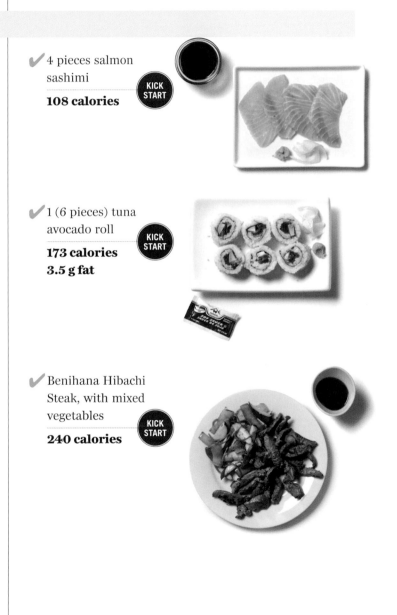

Chapter 13
SIDE DISHES

Side dishes are important for balancing your plate, adding variety, and making your meal more interesting and enjoyable. But as with almost all foods, it's important to pay attention to two things: how the dish is prepared and how big a portion you eat.

Let's talk first about potatoes, the most popular vegetable in the U.S. French fries and fad diets have given the potato a bad reputation that it doesn't deserve. Potatoes have plenty of fiber that fills you up, along with all-important vitamin C. I like baked potatoes best—I can control what goes with them, maybe just a dab of butter and a sprinkle of salt. (Beware, though: Restaurants sometimes coat potatoes with oil before baking, so even your "plain" baked potato may not be as healthy as you think!) Restaurants usually make mashed potatoes with butter and milk or cream to keep them moist, so I skip over those on the menu. And I try not to order fries because it's so hard to eat only a few (I just sneak from my daughters' plates)! I adore sweet potatoes, too. They have a gently sweet flavor, are naturally moist, and make a delicious snack. I sprinkle them with a bit of cinnamon and sugar.

Have you walked down the grains aisle lately? You'll be amazed at the variety of grains and grain mixes to choose from! Plain whole grains like quinoa, brown rice, wheat berries, and millet are incredibly filling. Their calories vary, but all are healthy, so I can't say one is better than the other. Grain mixes and pilafs cook faster than plain grains. But I always compare their sodium content—less is better—and use less oil or butter than the package calls for. The grain tastes just as good.

Eat beans! They have a lot of vitamins and minerals, fill you up, and are modest in calories. But you have to pay attention to what else is in them. Refried beans can be made with oil or lard—or they can have little or no fat, especially if you buy them canned. With baked beans, sugar and fat make the difference in calories. So read labels in the store and ask how the beans have been prepared in a restaurant.

I saved the best for last: vegetables. Such a plethora! When I don't have the time or patience to wash, peel, and chop veggies, I grab packages of fresh vegetables that are ready to go. Flavor with fresh herbs and other seasonings, rather than fat, and don't overlook the choices in the freezer section. At restaurants, ask for vegetables steamed or lightly sautéed, or have a side salad. Skip over any fried or heavily sauced options.

STOP EATING	START EATING
• Restaurant potato dishes like mashed potatoes, potatoes au gratin, and other dishes prepared or topped with butter, sour cream, cheese, or gravy	• A fist-sized baked potato, with a small bit of butter for flavor or with 0% Greek yogurt instead of sour cream
• Big orders of fries	• The smallest order of fries (or just one or two) and oven-baked fries at home
• Fatty or oily grain dishes such as fried rice, pasta in cream sauce, cheesy risotto, and some pilafs	• Whole grains such as brown rice, quinoa, wild rice, or bulgur wheat accented with seasonings, herbs, and flavorful vegetables
• Beans, particularly refried and baked, that are buried under high-calorie toppings (cheese, sour cream) or sugary sauces	• Fat-free or lightly seasoned beans, for example, fat-free refried beans or herbed limas
• Buttery or fatty vegetables such as buttered carrots, creamed spinach, tempura vegetables, onion rings, and fried zucchini	• Steamed or lightly sautéed vegetables

Side Dishes
POTATOES AND VEGETABLES

✖ STOP EATING | ✔ START EATING

🛒 *Packaged*

✖ ½ container Stouffer's Cheddar Potato Bake (270 calories, 17 g fat)

✖ 1 cup Alexia Harvest Sauté with Red Potatoes, Carrots, Green Beans, and Onions (240 calories, 16 g fat)

✖ ½ cup (½ box) Stouffer's Creamed Spinach (200 calories, 16 g fat)

✖ Idahoan Original Mashed Potatoes (180 calories)

✔ ⅔ cup Green Giant Steamers Broccoli & Cheese Sauce

KICK START

60 calories
2 g fat

✔ ½ cup Birds Eye Creamed Spinach

STEADY LOSS

90 calories
5 g fat

✔ 1 cup (⅕ box) Idahoan Au Gratin Homestyle Casserole

STEADY LOSS

150 calories

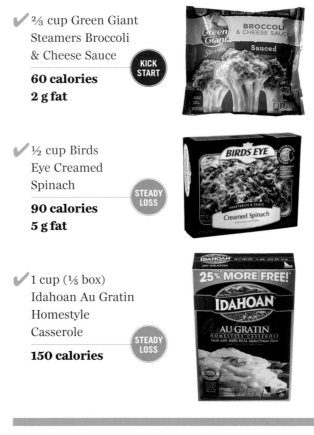

Other Good Choices

✔ ⅔ cup (1 container) Betty Crocker Microwavable Creamy Butter Mashed Potatoes **(80 calories, 1 g fat)**

✔ ½ cup Birds Eye Broccoli & Cheese Sauce **(90 calories, 5 g fat)**

✔ Betty Crocker Potatoes Au Gratin prepared from ½ cup (⅕ box) **(150 calories, 6 g fat)**

✔ 1 cup (from 1⅔ cup frozen) Birds Eye Steamfresh Chef's Favorites Roasted Red Potatoes & Green Beans **(120 calories, 2.5 g fat)**

✖ STOP EATING | ✔ START EATING

✗ *Restaurant*

✖ STOP EATING

✖ Palm Steakhouse Creamed Spinach (560 calories)

✖ Applebee's Loaded Baked Potato (400 calories, 23 g fat)

✖ Carrabba's Sauteed Broccoli and Cauliflower (317 calories, 31 g fat)

✖ Boston Market Loaded Mashed Potatoes (310 calories, 16 g fat)

✔ START EATING

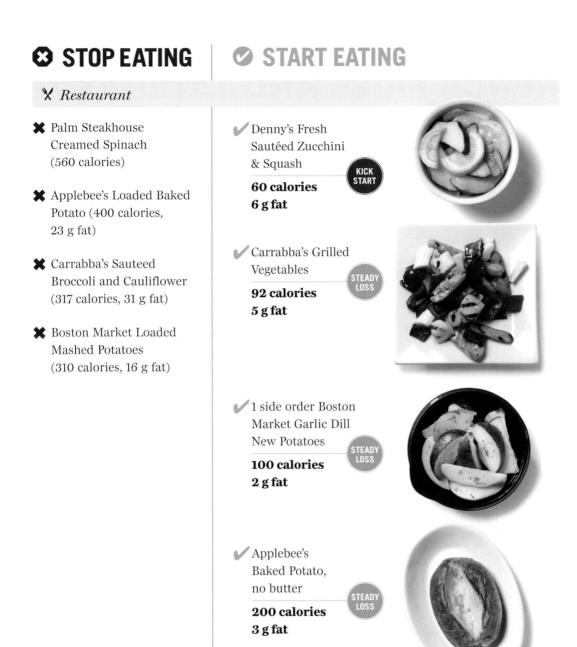

✔ Denny's Fresh Sautéed Zucchini & Squash

KICK START

60 calories
6 g fat

✔ Carrabba's Grilled Vegetables

STEADY LOSS

92 calories
5 g fat

✔ 1 side order Boston Market Garlic Dill New Potatoes

STEADY LOSS

100 calories
2 g fat

✔ Applebee's Baked Potato, no butter

STEADY LOSS

200 calories
3 g fat

Other Good Choices

✓ Chili's Steamed Broccoli (**40 calories, 0 g fat**)

✓ Boston Market Fresh Steamed Vegetables (**70 calories, 4 g fat**)

✓ TGI Friday's Fresh Spinach (**180 calories, 14 g fat**)

✓ Chili's Sweet Corn on the Cob (**190 calories, 7 g fat**)

✓ Wendy's Plain Baked Potato (**270 calories, 0 g fat**)

Side Dishes
FRENCH FRIES AND TATER TOTS

⊗ **STOP EATING**	⊘ **START EATING**

🛒 *Packaged*

✖ 14 pieces (½ carton) Ore-Ida Extra Crispy Easy Tater Tots Crispy Crowns (220 calories)

✖ 3 oz (¾ package) Ore-Ida Extra Crispy Easy Golden Fries (190 calories)

✔ 3 oz (⅕ package) Cascadian Farm Shoestring Fries **STEADY LOSS**
110 calories

✔ 3 oz (⅕ bag) Alexia Sweet Potato Fries with Sea Salt **STEADY LOSS**
140 calories

✔ 19 pieces (⅑ bag) Ore-Ida Mini Tater Tots **STEADY LOSS**
170 calories

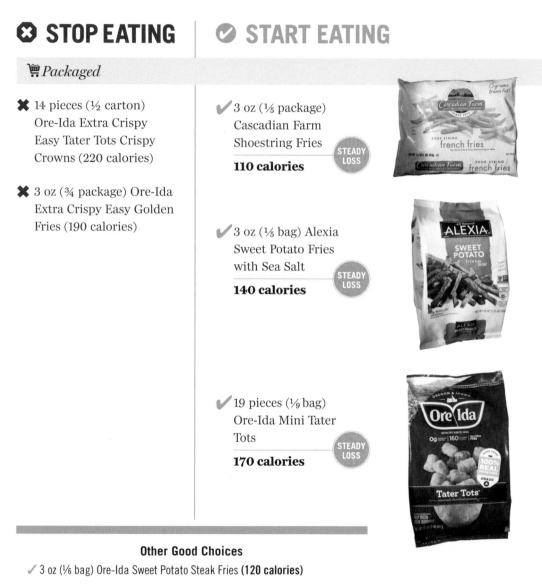

Other Good Choices

✓ 3 oz (⅙ bag) Ore-Ida Sweet Potato Steak Fries **(120 calories)**

✓ 3 oz (⅑ package) Alexia House Cut Fries with Sea Salt **(130 calories)**

✓ 3 oz (⅙ package) McCain 5 Minute Fries **(140 calories)**

✓ ⅔ cup (⅙ bag) Alexia Crispy Bite-Size Sweet Potato Puffs **(140 calories)**

✓ 3 oz (⅑ box) Ore-Ida Extra Crispy Fast Food Fries **(150 calories)**

⊗ STOP EATING | ✔ START EATING

✗ *Restaurant*

✗ Applebee's Chili Cheese Fries (630 calories, 33 g fat)

✗ Five Guys Little Fry (526 calories, 23 g fat)

✗ Large McDonald's French Fries (510 calories, 24 g fat)

✔ Mini Sonic Chili Cheese Natural-Cut Fries

STEADY LOSS

190 calories

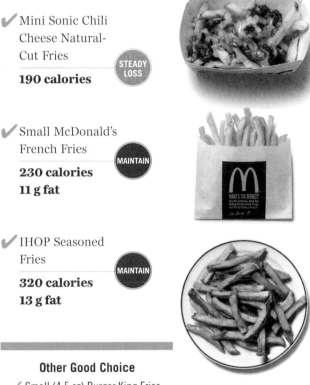

✔ Small McDonald's French Fries

MAINTAIN

230 calories
11 g fat

✔ IHOP Seasoned Fries

MAINTAIN

320 calories
13 g fat

Other Good Choice

✓ Small (4.5 oz) Burger King Fries (340 calories, 15 g fat)

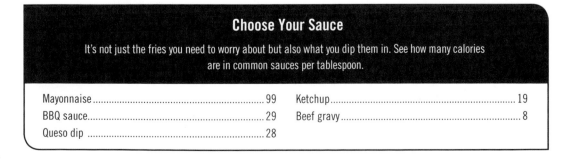

Choose Your Sauce

It's not just the fries you need to worry about but also what you dip them in. See how many calories are in common sauces per tablespoon.

Mayonnaise	99	Ketchup	19
BBQ sauce	29	Beef gravy	8
Queso dip	28		

Side Dishes
RICE AND OTHER GRAINS

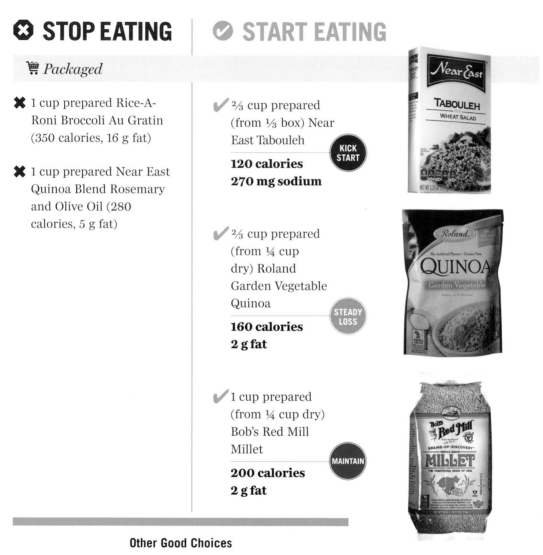

❌ STOP EATING	✅ START EATING

🛒 *Packaged*

❌ 1 cup prepared Rice-A-Roni Broccoli Au Gratin (350 calories, 16 g fat)

❌ 1 cup prepared Near East Quinoa Blend Rosemary and Olive Oil (280 calories, 5 g fat)

✓ ⅔ cup prepared (from ⅓ box) Near East Tabouleh — **KICK START**
120 calories
270 mg sodium

✓ ⅔ cup prepared (from ¼ cup dry) Roland Garden Vegetable Quinoa — **STEADY LOSS**
160 calories
2 g fat

✓ 1 cup prepared (from ¼ cup dry) Bob's Red Mill Millet — **MAINTAIN**
200 calories
2 g fat

Other Good Choices

✓ ⅓ cup dry (about ⅔ cup prepared) Fantastic World Foods Tabouli Salad Mix **(150 calories)**

✓ Roland Mediterranean Quinoa **(170 calories)**

✓ 1 cup prepared Near East Original Plain Wheat Couscous **(180 calories)**

✓ Uncle Ben's Ready Rice Rice Pilaf **(210 calories, 2.5 g fat)**

❌ STOP EATING | ✔ START EATING

❌ TGI Friday's Jasmine Rice Pilaf (420 calories, 11 g fat)

❌ Panda Express White Steamed Rice (380 calories, 0 g fat)

❌ PF Chang's Brown Rice (310 calories, 2 g fat)

✔ Red Lobster Wild Rice Pilaf

STEADY LOSS

170 calories
3 g fat

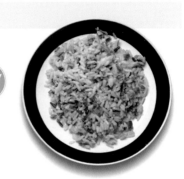

✔ ½ order Panda Express Brown Steamed Rice

STEADY LOSS

210 calories
2 g fat

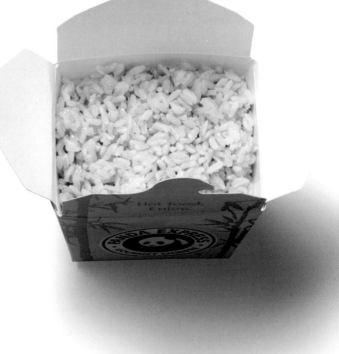

Choose Your Toppings

Wondering if it's really worth it to switch to brown rice or another ancient grain? See how many calories are in each per ½ cup cooked.

Amaranth	125
Kamut	114
Quinoa	111
Brown rice	108
Millet	104
White rice	103
Wild rice	82
Buckwheat	77

Side Dishes
BEANS

❌ STOP EATING	✅ START EATING

🛒 *Packaged*

STOP EATING

❌ ½ cup Bush's Best Country Style Baked Beans (160 calories)

❌ ½ cup Goya Traditional Refried Pinto Beans (140 calories)

START EATING

✔ ½ cup Old El Paso Black Bean Refried Beans

KICK START

100 calories

✔ ½ cup Bush's Best Vegetarian Baked Beans

KICK START

130 calories

✔ ½ cup Pacific Organic Refried Black Beans with Green Chilies

KICK START

130 calories
1.5 g fat

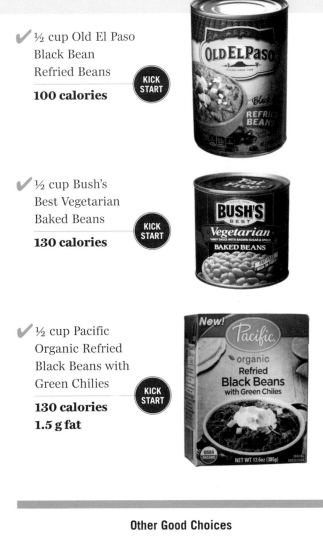

Other Good Choices

✓ ½ cup Old El Paso Traditional Refried Beans (**110 calories**)

✓ ½ cup Eden Organic Refried Black Beans (**110 calories**)

✓ ½ cup Ortega Vegetarian Refried Beans (**120 calories**)

❌ STOP EATING | ✅ START EATING

✖ El Pollo Loco Pinto Beans (200 calories)

✖ Taco Bell Pintos 'n Cheese (190 calories)

✔ Taco Bell Black Beans

KICK START

80 calories

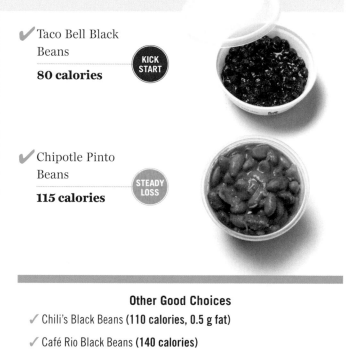

✔ Chipotle Pinto Beans

STEADY LOSS

115 calories

Other Good Choices

✓ Chili's Black Beans **(110 calories, 0.5 g fat)**

✓ Café Rio Black Beans **(140 calories)**

✓ Café Rio Pinto Beans **(150 calories, 2.5 g fat)**

Chapter 14
APPETIZERS AND SNACKS

It's too hard to go more than a few hours without eating, especially when you're trying to lose weight. Snacks and appetizers help keep me from over-eating at mealtime. Fresh fruits and vegetables are my go-to snacks. They're quick, easy, full of vitamins and fiber, and low in calories. If I'm in the mood for something more filling, I'll often opt for a minimeal, such as a small cup of soup or a few slices of deli turkey and cheese.

I was shocked by the diet damage that can be done by appetizers in restaurants. For example, a full order of wings at Outback Steakhouse has nearly 1200 calories—as much as you'll have on an entire Kickstart day! (You're supposed to share the wings, but I have friends who keep them all to themselves.) The key with all these foods? Portion control. Enjoy a few bites, then move on to foods that will fill you up and fit better into your eating plan.

Most restaurant appetizers are designed to be shared. So if you must indulge while on the Stop & Drop Diet, split them with at least three other people—or, in the case, of those Outback wings, a whole tableful!—or have just a small portion and box up the rest. (One exception I love is shrimp cocktail. Eight jumbo shrimp have only 40 calories! Add another 20 or so for a tablespoon of cocktail sauce and there's still room for a small glass of wine. Just stay away from fried shrimp and creamy dressings like tartar sauce.) Ask the waiter to take away the bread basket or at least to not refill it. You could easily add a few hundred calories to your meal by mindlessly munching on a few breadsticks or rolls.

When picking up or preparing snacks at home or on the go, look for smaller packages for built-in portion control. Even then, though, I can't stress enough how important it is to read labels. Hummus, for instance, is one of my favorite dips; it's creamy, delicious, and fills me up with protein and fiber. I was happy to see a single-serve cup from one of my favorite brands, Sabra, until I turned it over to look at the nutrition label and saw that one serving packed 260 calories and 19 g fat. Plus, if I ate the pretzels that came with the cup, that would add another 120 calories and 1 g fat. No, thank you! Instead, I buy the family-size carton and portion it into smaller containers to bring to work.

Similarly, I love guacamole—bring on the MUFAs!—but I always pay attention to portion size because it's pretty concentrated in calories. For creamy dips, as with creamy dressings, 0% Greek yogurt is my secret weapon. Not many calories and plenty of protein and calcium, so what could be bad? Use it to make your favorite onion or spinach dip, or buy brands that already have a Greek yogurt base, and you'll drop calories big-time. And for dipping, I always go for the vegetables first. Even pita, veggie, and healthier chips pack a wallop of calories and are easy to overeat.

When you're looking for healthy snacks, the popcorn aisle is a great place to go. I've given you a head start on microwave and already popped brands that are lower in fat and calories. On the other hand, nuts, chocolates, dried fruit, and cheeses have pluses and minuses. They're packed with tummy-trimming ingredients such as MUFAs, protein, fiber, and calcium, but they also have a fair number of calories in a relatively small portion. So again, pay attention to the portions we recommend, and take time to enjoy them. (Wondering how to split portions of something with multiple components, like the Starbucks Cheese & Fruit Bistro Box? Just eat about half of each component—i.e., half the cheese, half the fruit, half the nuts, and half the crackers.)

STOP EATING	START EATING
• Full orders of appetizers	• A small portion of an appetizer order for the table
• Big portions of fatty dips like onion dip, spinach-artichoke dip, hot crab dip	• Modest portions of healthy dips like hummus and guacamole, and dips made with Greek yogurt
• All sorts of chips for dipping, including pita chips	• Fresh veggie dippers
• Fried or popcorn shrimp	• Shrimp cocktail
• Buttery popcorn, especially from movie theaters	• DIY light microwave popcorn, or ready-popped light varieties
• Oversized bags of chocolate and nut trail mix	• A 100-calorie bag of chocolate, dried fruit, nuts, or trail mix

Appetizers and Snacks
MIDDLE EASTERN DIPS

⊗ STOP EATING | ⊘ START EATING

🛒 *Packaged*

✖ California Pizza Kitchen Tuscan Hummus with wheat whole grain pita (970 calories, 33 g fat)

✖ Sabra Classic Hummus with Pretzels (380 calories, 20 g fat)

✖ Au Bon Pain Hummus & Pita Chip Snack Pack (340 calories, 21 g fat)

✔ 2 Tbsp (1 oz) Cento Eggplant Appetizer

18 calories · KICK START

✔ 2 Tbsp (1 oz) Marco Polo Caponata

40 calories · KICK START

✔ 2 Tbsp (1 oz) Athenos Roasted Red Pepper Hummus

60 calories · KICK START

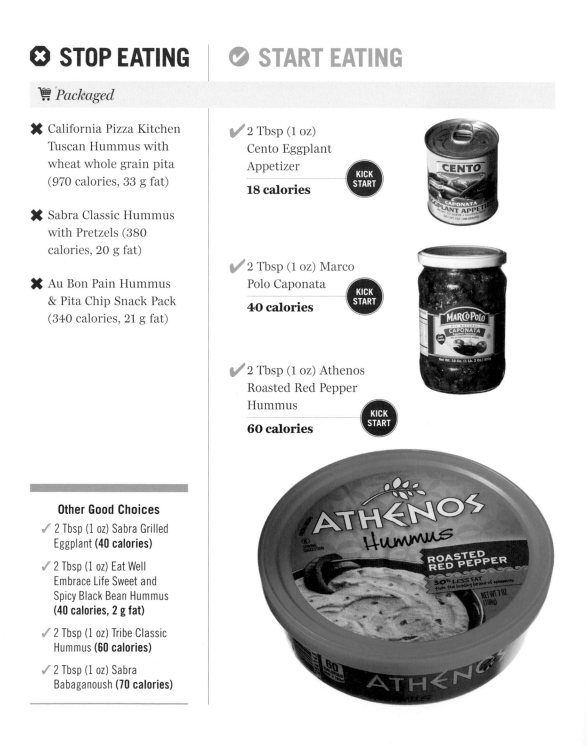

Other Good Choices

✓ 2 Tbsp (1 oz) Sabra Grilled Eggplant (**40 calories**)

✓ 2 Tbsp (1 oz) Eat Well Embrace Life Sweet and Spicy Black Bean Hummus (**40 calories, 2 g fat**)

✓ 2 Tbsp (1 oz) Tribe Classic Hummus (**60 calories**)

✓ 2 Tbsp (1 oz) Sabra Babaganoush (**70 calories**)

✅ START EATING

🛒 *Packaged*

✔ 2 Tbsp (1 oz) Eat Well Embrace Life Wasabi Edamame Hummus

60 calories
4.5 g fat

KICK START

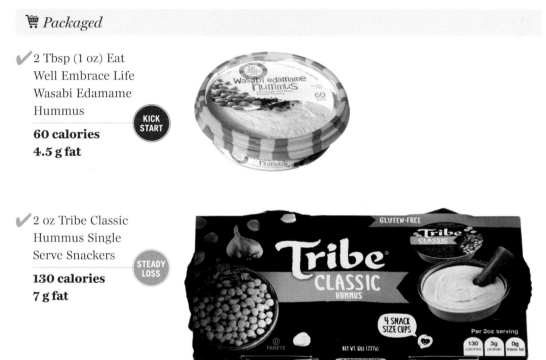

✔ 2 oz Tribe Classic Hummus Single Serve Snackers

130 calories
7 g fat

STEADY LOSS

Choose Your Dippers

What you use as a vehicle for your dips can make a big difference. See how many calories are in your favorite dippers.

11 (1 oz) whole wheat pita chips 130	5 broccoli florets 15
Small (4 inch) whole wheat pita, cut into wedges...... 74	5 cherry tomatoes.. 15
20 thin pretzel sticks................................... 42	2 celery stalks 13
10 baby carrots....................................... 35	

Appetizers and Snacks
CREAMY DIPS

❌ **STOP EATING**	✅ **START EATING**

🏠 *Homemade*

❌ ¼ cup homemade onion dip made with Lipton Recipe Secrets Onion Dip Mix and mayonnaise (410 calories, 11 g fat)

✓ ¼ cup homemade onion dip made with Lipton Recipe Secrets Onion Dip Mix and plain 0% Greek yogurt

KICK START

54 calories
0 g fat

HOW TO MAKE IT

Combine 1 packet Lipton Recipe Secrets Onion Dip Mix with 2 cups plain 0% Greek yogurt. (Makes 8 servings)

🛒 *Packaged*

❌ 2 Tbsp Marzetti Spinach Veggie Dip (110 calories)

❌ 2 Tbsp Robert Rothschild Farm Artichoke Spinach Dip (70 calories)

✓ 2 Tbsp Cedar's Cucumber Dill Garlic Tzatziki

STEADY LOSS

40 calories

Other Good Choice

✓ 2 Tbsp Sabra Cucumber Dill Greek Yogurt Dip **(40 calories)**

✓ 2 Tbsp Marzetti Otria Garden Herb Ranch Greek Yogurt Dip **(60 calories)**

✓ 2 Tbsp Frito-Lay French Onion Dip

STEADY LOSS

60 calories

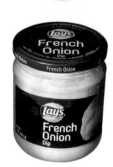

❌ STOP EATING | ✅ START EATING

❌ Applebee's Spinach & Artichoke Dip with tortilla chips (1390 calories, 94 g fat)

❌ California Pizza Kitchen Spinach Artichoke Dip with tortilla chips (930 calories, 51 g fat)

✔ Cosi Spinach & Artichoke Dip with bread

336 calories
11 g fat

(MAINTAIN)

Choose Your Base

Which creamy base you choose for your dip mix makes a big difference in calories. Here are calories per 2 tablespoons for common dip bases.

Mayonnaise	198
Light mayonnaise	71
Sour cream	46
Light sour cream	42
Plain low-fat yogurt	19
Plain 0% Greek yogurt	17
Plain fat-free yogurt	17

Choose Your Dippers

What you use as a vehicle for your dips can make a big difference. See how many calories are in your favorite dippers.

1 piece Cosi multigrain flatbread	235
10 (1 oz) Food Should Taste Good Multigrain Tortilla Chips	140
16 (1 oz) Pringles Reduced Fat Crisps	140
11 (1 oz) whole wheat pita chips	130
3 thin slices (1 oz) Italian bread	81
Small (4 inch) whole wheat pita, cut into wedges	74
20 thin pretzel sticks	42

MEXICAN DIPS AND NACHOS

❌ STOP EATING | ✅ START EATING

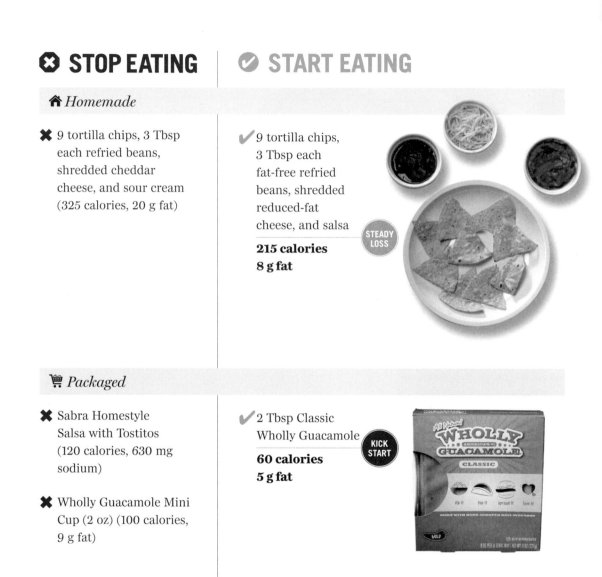

🏠 *Homemade*

❌ 9 tortilla chips, 3 Tbsp each refried beans, shredded cheddar cheese, and sour cream (325 calories, 20 g fat)

✅ 9 tortilla chips, 3 Tbsp each fat-free refried beans, shredded reduced-fat cheese, and salsa

STEADY LOSS

**215 calories
8 g fat**

🛒 *Packaged*

❌ Sabra Homestyle Salsa with Tostitos (120 calories, 630 mg sodium)

❌ Wholly Guacamole Mini Cup (2 oz) (100 calories, 9 g fat)

✅ 2 Tbsp Classic Wholly Guacamole

KICK START

**60 calories
5 g fat**

Other Good Choices

✓ 2 Tbsp Santa Barbara Pico de Gallo Salsa (**10 calories**)

✓ 2 Tbsp Santa Barbara Garden Style Salsa (**15 calories**)

✓ 2 Tbsp Newman's Own Peach Salsa (**25 calories**)

✓ 2 Tbsp Tostitos Salsa con Queso (**40 calories, 2.5 g fat**)

❌ STOP EATING | ✅ START EATING

✗ *Restaurant*

❌ Chili's Tableside Guacamole (1490 calories, 97 g fat)

❌ Applebee's Queso Blanco (1050 calories, 72 g fat)

❌ Taco Bell Nachos BellGrande (760 calories, 38 g fat)

Other Good Choices

✓ Del Taco Chili Cheese Nachos **(260 calories, 6 g fat)**

✓ Taco Bell Triple Layer Nachos **(320 calories, 15 g fat)**

✓ California Pizza Kitchen White Corn Guacamole & Chips **(410 calories, 22 g fat)**

✓ ¼ order Ruby Tuesday Queso & Chips

288 calories
18 g fat

STEADY LOSS

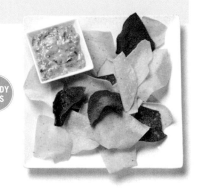

✓ ¼ order Chili's Classic Nachos, no chicken or beef topping

300 calories

STEADY LOSS

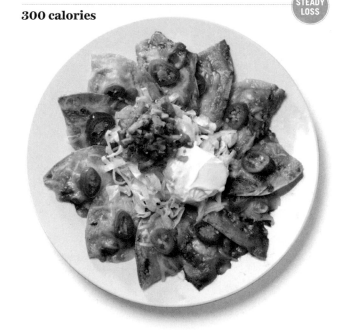

Choose Your Chips

Different styles of tortilla chips give you slightly different calories. Here are some to consider.

7 (1 oz) Tostitos Cantina Traditional Tortilla Chips 150	1 oz Popcorners Sea Salt 130
10 (1 oz) Food Should Taste Good Multigrain Tortilla Chip 140	8 (1 oz) Snyder's of Hanover Restaurant Style Tortilla Chips 130
10 (1 oz) Food Should Taste Good Blue Corn Tortilla Chips 140	19 (1 oz) Garden of Eatin' Baked Yellow Tortilla Chips 120

Appetizers and Snacks
WINGS

✖ STOP EATING | ✔ START EATING

🛒 *Packaged*

✖ 3 pieces (3 oz) Banquet Hot & Spicy Wings (240 calories)

✔ 3 (5 oz) TGI Friday's Chicken Wings Buffalo Style Sauce   **STEADY LOSS**

180 calories

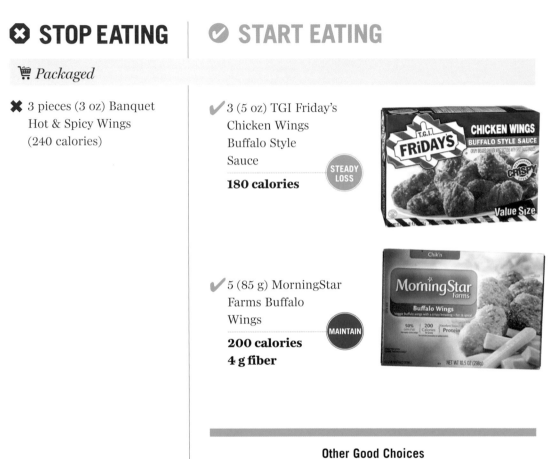

✔ 5 (85 g) MorningStar Farms Buffalo Wings   **MAINTAIN**

200 calories
4 g fiber

Other Good Choices

✔ 3 pieces (3 oz) Tyson Buffalo Style Boneless Chicken Wyngz **(150 calories)**

✔ 3 oz (about ⅓ package) Tyson Any'tizers Grillin' Wings Rotisserie Flavored Wings **(180 calories, 11 g fat)**

❌ STOP EATING | ✅ START EATING

✗ *Restaurant*

✖ Chili's Boneless Buffalo Wings (1090 calories, 73 g fat)

✖ Ruby Tuesday Fire Wings (712 calories, 44 g fat)

Other Good Choices

✓ 1 Bertucci's Grilled Tuscan Wing **(66 calories, 5 g fat)**

✓ 1 KFC Hot Wing **(70 calories, 4 g fat)**

Choose Your Dressing

Slight variations in blue cheese dressing can add up to big differences in calories. See how many calories there are per tablespoon in different dressings.

Chunky blue cheese dip.........80
Blue cheese dressing............73
Light chunky blue cheese
  dip.......................................40
Fat-free blue cheese
  dressing..............................20

✔ 1 Applebee's Boneless Wing (about ⅛ order), with celery and 1 Tbsp dressing

STEADY LOSS

103 calories
5.5 g fat

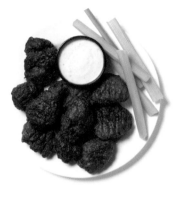

✔ 2 Ruby Tuesday Fire Wings (about ¼ order), with celery

KICK START

178 calories
11 g fat

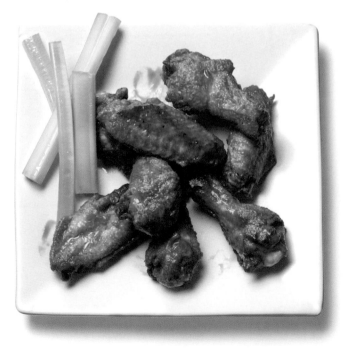

Appetizers and Snacks
SHRIMP

✖ STOP EATING	✔ START EATING

🏠 *Homemade*

✖ 8 large shrimp with ¼ cup tartar sauce (167 calories, 11 g fat)

✔ 8 large shrimp, with ¼ cup cocktail sauce

115 calories
2 g fat

KICK START

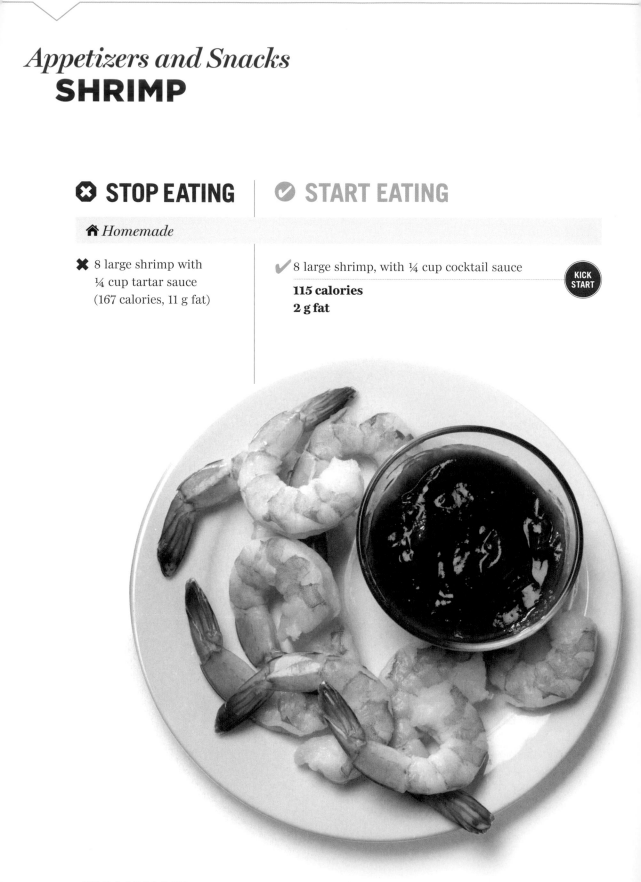

✖ STOP EATING | ✔ START EATING

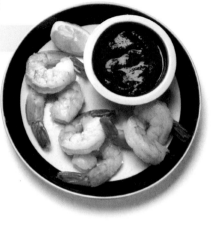

✖ Restaurant

✖ Longhorn Steakhouse
Wild West Shrimp, with
ranch dressing (1030
calories, 80 g fat)

✖ Legal Sea Food Buffalo
Popcorn Shrimp (740
calories)

✖ Red Lobster Parrot Isle
Jumbo Coconut Shrimp
(510 calories, 34 g fat)

✔ Red Lobster
Signature Shrimp
Cocktail

KICK START

**100 calories
0.5 g fat**

✔ Full order Longhorn
Steakhouse Redrock
Grilled Shrimp, no
sauce

KICK START

**160 calories
3 g fat**

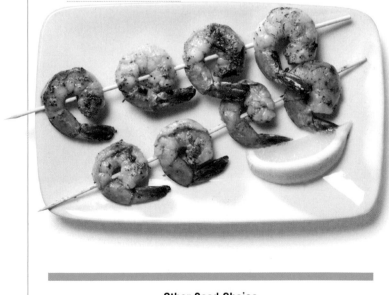

Other Good Choice

✓ Legal Sea Food Jumbo Shrimp Cocktail **(199 calories)**

EGG ROLLS, SPRING ROLLS, POTSTICKERS, AND WONTONS

❌ STOP EATING | ✅ START EATING

🛒 *Packaged*

STOP EATING:

❌ 4 Annie Chun's Spicy Vegetable Mini Wontons (240 calories)

❌ 7 Annie Chun's Organic Shiitake & Vegetable Potstickers (240 calories)

START EATING:

✔ 4 (⅙ package) Annie Chun's Chicken & Cilantro Mini Wontons

KICK START

50 calories

✔ 1 Van Low Fat Vegetable Egg Roll with sauce

STEADY LOSS

120 calories

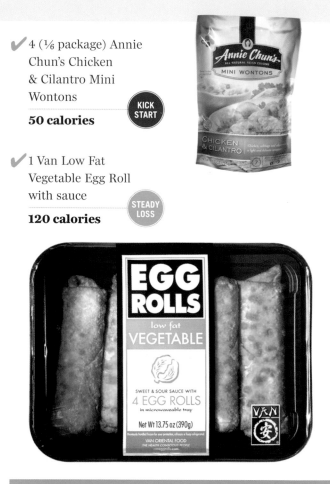

Other Good Choices

✔ 3 InnovAsian Chicken Shumai Dumplings, with sauce **(130 calories)**

✔ 2 (¼ package) Ling Ling Mini Vegetable Spring Rolls with sauce **(140 calories)**

✔ 4 (⅓ package) Cohen's Vegetable Egg Rolls **(150 calories)**

✖ STOP EATING | ✓ START EATING

✗ Restaurant

✖ Chili's Southwestern Eggrolls (800 calories, 2180 mg sodium)

✖ 2 Pei Wei Pork Egg Rolls with sauce (510 calories, 1680 mg sodium)

✓ 2 Panda Express Veggie Spring Rolls **KICK START**

160 calories
520 mg sodium

✓ 2 PF Chang's Vegetable Spring Rolls, no sauce **MAINTAIN**

210 calories
860 mg sodium

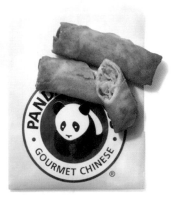

Choose Your Sauce

Hot sauces tend to be lower in calories than other dipping sauces. See how many calories are in common Asian sauces per tablespoon.

Peanut sauce	46
Duck sauce	40
Chili garlic sauce	15
Horseradish mustard	15
Soy sauce	8

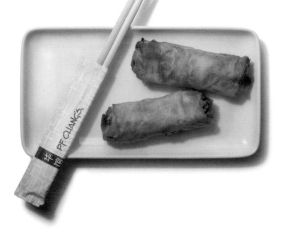

Other Good Choices

✓ Panda Express Chicken Potstickers **(160 calories)**

✓ ½ order Applebee's Grilled Chicken Wonton Tacos **(230 calories)**

Appetizers and Snacks
BREAD AND ROLLS

✖ STOP EATING	✔ START EATING

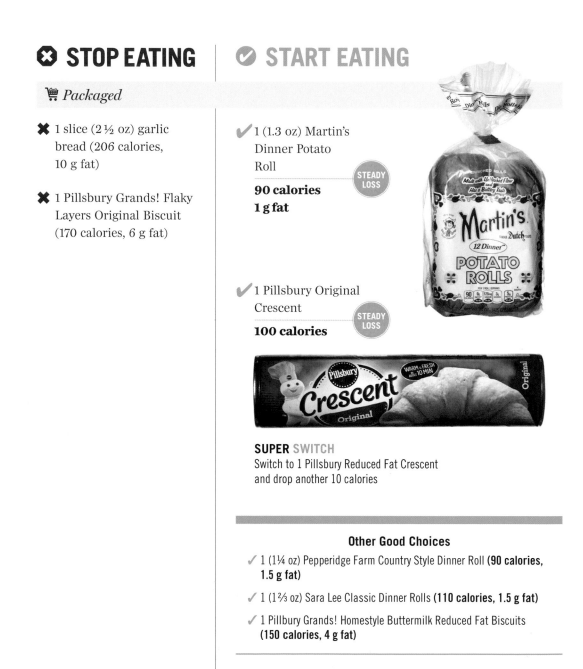

✖ STOP EATING

🛒 *Packaged*

✖ 1 slice (2 ½ oz) garlic bread (206 calories, 10 g fat)

✖ 1 Pillsbury Grands! Flaky Layers Original Biscuit (170 calories, 6 g fat)

✔ START EATING

✔ 1 (1.3 oz) Martin's Dinner Potato Roll — **STEADY LOSS**

90 calories
1 g fat

✔ 1 Pillsbury Original Crescent — **STEADY LOSS**

100 calories

SUPER SWITCH
Switch to 1 Pillsbury Reduced Fat Crescent and drop another 10 calories

---

Other Good Choices

✓ 1 (1¼ oz) Pepperidge Farm Country Style Dinner Roll (**90 calories, 1.5 g fat**)

✓ 1 (1⅔ oz) Sara Lee Classic Dinner Rolls (**110 calories, 1.5 g fat**)

✓ 1 Pillbury Grands! Homestyle Buttermilk Reduced Fat Biscuits (**150 calories, 4 g fat**)

✖ STOP EATING | ✔ START EATING

✖ 1 order Olive Garden Bruschetta Caprese (660 calories, 8 g sugars)

✖ 1 (3.3 oz) Bob Evans brioche bun (277 calories, 7 g sugars)

✖ 1 piece Cosi multigrain bread (235 calories, 3 g sugars)

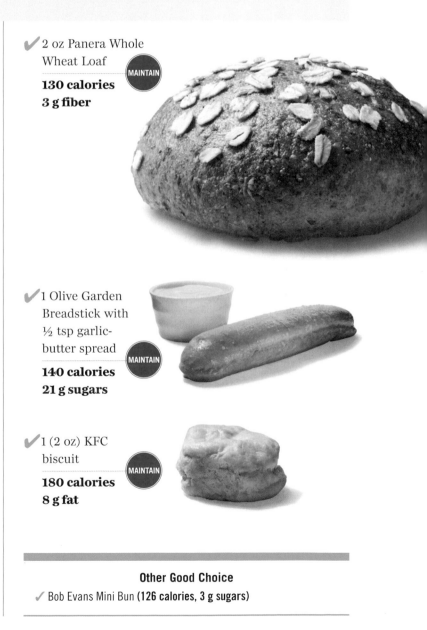

✔ 2 oz Panera Whole Wheat Loaf **MAINTAIN**
130 calories
3 g fiber

✔ 1 Olive Garden Breadstick with ½ tsp garlic-butter spread **MAINTAIN**
140 calories
21 g sugars

✔ 1 (2 oz) KFC biscuit **MAINTAIN**
180 calories
8 g fat

Choose Your Roll

Beware the breadbasket! It can easily add 100 or more calories to your dinner, especially if you eat more than one. See how many calories are in different types of rolls.

Biscuit (2 oz)	170
Whole wheat pita (6 inch)	170
Kaiser roll (2 oz)	167
Brown and serve club roll (1¾ oz)	130
Potato roll (1¾ oz)	120
Crescent roll (1 oz)	100
Egg dinner roll (1¼ oz)	107
Whole wheat dinner roll (1¼ oz)	96

Other Good Choice
✓ Bob Evans Mini Bun (126 calories, 3 g sugars)

Appetizers and Snacks
PRETZELS

⊗ STOP EATING	⊘ START EATING

🛒 *Packaged*

✖ Kim & Scott's Traditional Bavarian Pretzel (450 calories)

✖ 1 pouch (½ package) Lean Cuisine Three Cheese & Spinach Stuffed Pretzels (220 calories)

Other Good Choices

✓ 11 (1 oz) Snack Factory Pretzel Crisps Original (**110 calories**)

✓ 10 (1 oz) Trader Joe's Peanut Butter Filled Pretzels (**127 calories**)

✓ 9 (1 oz) Snyder's of Hanover Peanut Butter Pretzel Sandwiches (**130 calories**)

✓ 2 SuperPretzel Pretzelfils Mozzarella (**130 calories**)

✓ ⅓ cup (1 oz) Snyder's of Hanover Honey Mustard & Onion Pretzel Pieces (**140 calories**)

✔ 20 (1 oz) Snyder's of Hanover Mini Pretzels **KICK START**
110 calories

✔ 7 (1 oz) Herr's Whole Grain Honey Wheat Pretzel Sticks **KICK START**
110 calories

✔ 4 (1 oz) Snack Factory Pretzel Crisps Peanut Butter Crunch **STEADY LOSS**
140 calories

✔ 1 pouch (½ package) Lean Cuisine Culinary Collection Monterey Jack Jalapeño Stuffed Pretzels **STEADY LOSS**
190 calories

❌ STOP EATING | ✅ START EATING

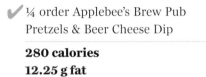

✗ Restaurant

✗ Full order TGI Friday's Warm Pretzels with Craft Beer-Cheese Dipping Sauce (1180 calories, 60 g fat)

✔ ¼ order Applebee's Brew Pub Pretzels & Beer Cheese Dip

MAINTAIN

280 calories
12.25 g fat

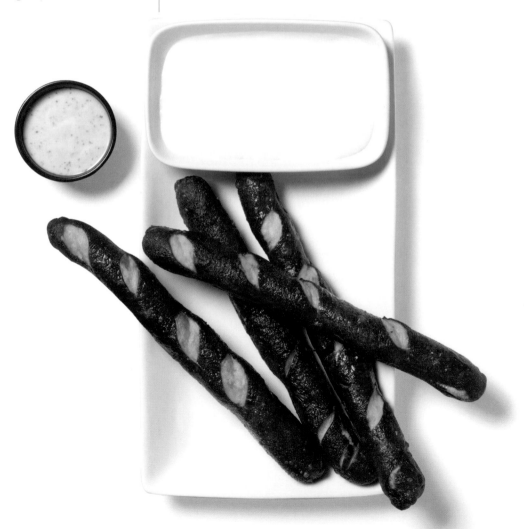

Appetizers and Snacks
POTATO, CORN, AND VEGGIE CHIPS

❌ STOP EATING | ✅ START EATING

🛒 Packaged

❌ 32 (1 oz) Fritos The Original Corn Chips (160 calories)

❌ 15 (1 oz) Lay's Classic Potato Chips (160 calories)

❌ 16 (1 oz) Pringles The Original (150 calories)

❌ 14 (1 oz) Terra Original Chips (150 calories)

❌ 7 (1 oz) Tostitos Cantina Traditional Tortilla Chips (150 calories)

✓ 1 oz bag Popcorners Twisted Salt Popped Whole Grain Chips

KICK START

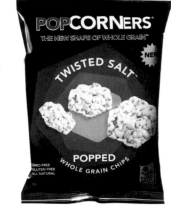

Other Good Choices

✓ 15 (1 oz) Pringles Original Fat Free Potato Chips **(70 calories)**

✓ 9 (1 oz) Ruffles Baked! Original Potato Crisps **(120 calories)**

✓ 20 (1 oz) Kettle Brand Sea Salt Real Sliced Potatoes Potato Chips **(120 calories)**

✓ 80 (1 oz) Good Health Veggie Stix **(120 calories)**

✓ 23 (1 oz) Popchips Sea Salt Potato Chips **(120 calories)**

✓ 19 (1 oz) Garden of Eatin' Baked Yellow Tortilla Chips **(120 calories)**

✓ 10 (1 oz) Food Should Taste Good Multi-Grain Tortilla Chips **(140 calories)**

✓ 1.1 oz bag Popcorners Sea Salt Popped Corn Chips **(140 calories)**

✔ START EATING

🛒 *Packaged*

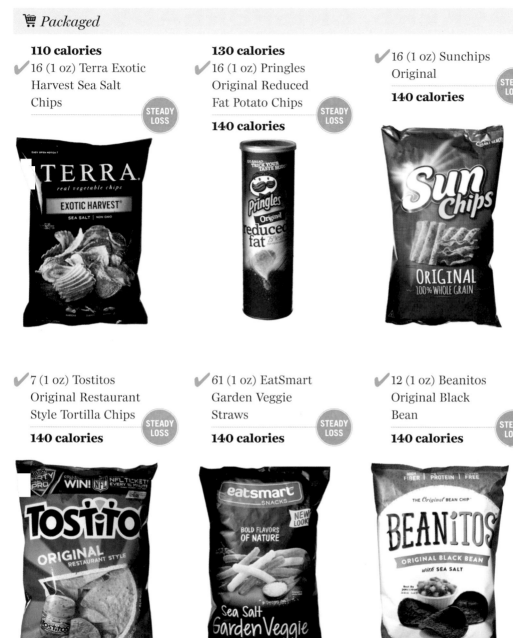

110 calories
✔ 16 (1 oz) Terra Exotic Harvest Sea Salt Chips — STEADY LOSS

130 calories
✔ 16 (1 oz) Pringles Original Reduced Fat Potato Chips — STEADY LOSS

140 calories

✔ 16 (1 oz) Sunchips Original — STEADY LOSS

140 calories

✔ 7 (1 oz) Tostitos Original Restaurant Style Tortilla Chips — STEADY LOSS

140 calories

✔ 61 (1 oz) EatSmart Garden Veggie Straws — STEADY LOSS

140 calories

✔ 12 (1 oz) Beanitos Original Black Bean — STEADY LOSS

140 calories

Appetizers and Snacks
CRACKERS, CRISPBREADS, AND PITA CHIPS

❌ STOP EATING	✓ START EATING

🏠 *Homemade*

❌ Pita chips made with a regular 6-inch pita brushed with 1 Tbsp oil (300 calories, 14 g fat)

✓ Pita chips made with 1 oz whole wheat pita and cooking spray

92 calories

STEADY LOSS

HOW TO MAKE IT

Split 1 oz pita in half to make two rounds and cut into 6 wedges each. Spray with a couple sprays of cooking oil. Bake at 350°F until crisp, about 10 minutes. (Makes 1 serving)

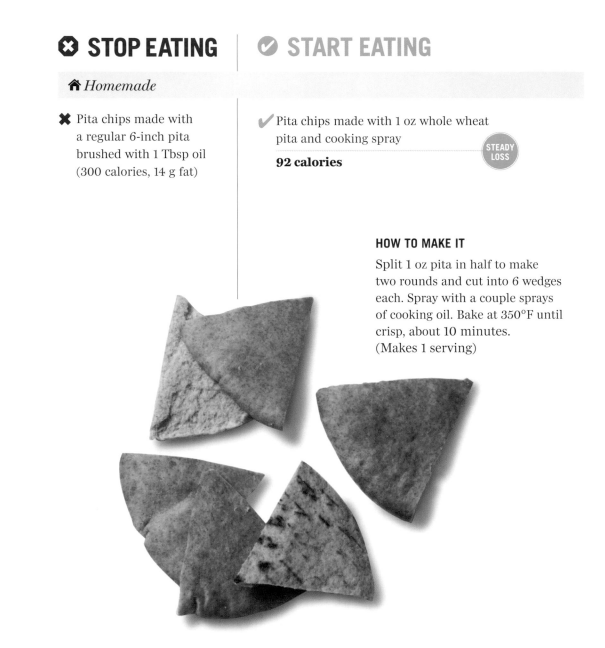

❌ STOP EATING | ✅ START EATING

🛒 *Packaged*

❌ 16 (1 oz) Wheat Thins Hint of Salt (150 calories)

❌ 15 (1 oz) Triscuit Thin Crisps (130 calories)

❌ 10 (1 oz) Stacy's Simply Naked Pita Chips (130 calories)

✅ 1 piece (15 g) Wasa Fiber Crispbread **(KICK START)**

40 calories
2.5 g fiber

✅ 8 (15 g) Keebler Town House Sea Salt & Olive Oil Flatbread Crisps **(KICK START)**

70 calories

✅ 6 (1 oz) Reduced Fat Triscuit crackers **(KICK START)**

110 calories

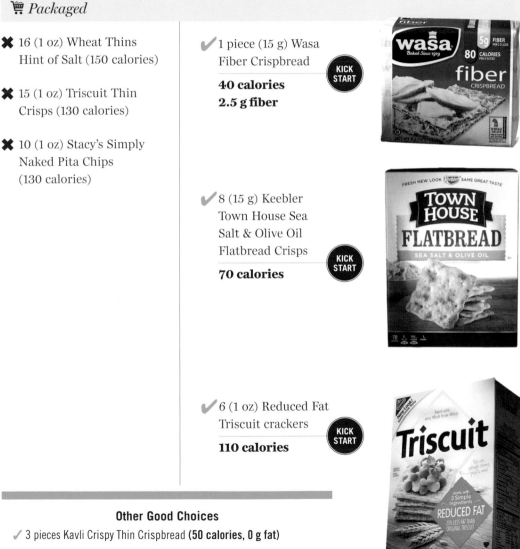

Other Good Choices

✓ 3 pieces Kavli Crispy Thin Crispbread **(50 calories, 0 g fat)**

✓ 3 pieces Finn Crisp Original **(66 calories, 0.5 g fat)**

✓ 15 (1 oz) Wheat Thins Fiber Selects Garden Vegetables **(120 calories, 4 g fat)**

Appetizers and Snacks
POPCORN AND CHEESE PUFFS

⊗ **STOP EATING**	⊘ **START EATING**

🛒 *Packaged*

STOP EATING

✖ 4 cups Wise All Natural Popcorn (300 calories, 18 g fat, 400 mg sodium)

✖ 3 cups Smartfood Sweet & Salty Kettle Corn (280 calories, 12 g fat, 22 g sugars)

✖ 21 (1 oz) Crunchy Cheetos (150 calories, 10 g fat)

START EATING

✔ 1½ Tbsp (about ¼ bag) unpopped Orville Redenbacher's SmartPop! Butter

60 calories

KICK START

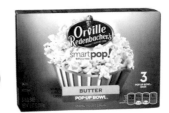

✔ 2 Tbsp (about ½ bag) unpopped Jolly Time Crispy 'n White Light

120 calories

KICK START

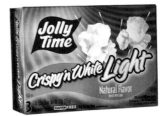

SUPER SWITCH
Switch to Jolly Time Yellow Kernels and drop another 10 calories

Other Good Choices

✓ 2 Tbsp (about ½ bag) unpopped Jollytime Healthy Pop Kettle Corn **(110 calories)**

✓ 4 cups (1 oz) Angie's Boom Chicka Pop Sea Salt Popcorn **(140 calories)**

✓ 4 cups (1 oz) Wise Reduced Fat Butter Popcorn **(140 calories)**

✓ 3 cups Pop Secret Pre-Popped Kettle Corn **(150 calories)**

✓ START EATING

🛒 *Packaged*

✓ ½ cup (1 oz) Cracker Jack Original Caramel Coated Popcorn & Peanuts

120 calories — KICK START

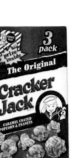

✓ 3 ¼ cups (1 oz) Angie's Boom Chicka Pop Lightly Sweet Popcorn

120 calories — KICK START

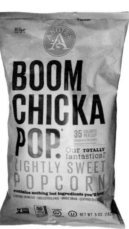

✓ 3 ¾ cups Skinny Pop Original Popcorn

150 calories — STEADY LOSS

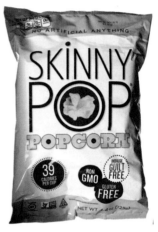

✓ 34 (1 oz) Cheetos Oven Baked Crunchy Cheese Flavored Snack

130 calories — STEADY LOSS

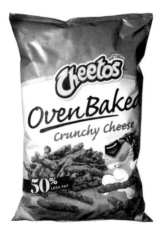

✓ 1 oz (less than ¼ bag) Pirate's Booty Smart Puffs Real Cheddar

140 calories — MAINTAIN

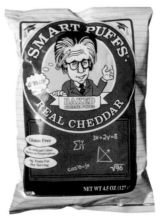

NUTS, CHOCOLATES, AND DRIED FRUIT

✖ STOP EATING | ✔ START EATING

🛒 *Packaged*

STOP EATING

✖ 1.5 oz Planters Daybreak Blend Berry Almond Go-Pak (180 calories, 7 g fat)

✖ 1 bag (1.69 oz) M&M's milk chocolate (240 calories)

✖ 1 (1.55 oz) Hershey's Cookies 'n' Crème Bar (220 calories)

✖ ¼ cup Planters Nutrition Energy Mix (190 calories, 15 g fat)

✖ 3 Twix Caramel Cookie Bars Mini (whole package) (150 calories, 15 g sugars)

START EATING

✔ 1 Reese's Dark Peanut Butter Cup Miniature — **KICK START**

44 calories
4.2 g sugars

✔ Ghirardelli Milk & Caramel square — **KICK START**

60 calories
3 g sugars

✔ 1 oz box Sun-Maid raisins — **KICK START**

90 calories
0 g fat

⊘ START EATING

🛒 *Packaged*

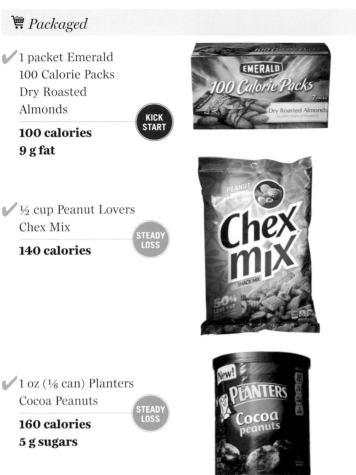

✔ 1 packet Emerald 100 Calorie Packs Dry Roasted Almonds

KICK START

100 calories
9 g fat

✔ ½ cup Peanut Lovers Chex Mix

STEADY LOSS

140 calories

✔ 1 oz (⅙ can) Planters Cocoa Peanuts

STEADY LOSS

160 calories
5 g sugars

Other Good Choices

✔ ¼ cup Sahale Snacks Premium Blend Maple Pecans (**150 calories, 10 g fat**)

✔ ¼ cup Planters Fruit & Nut Trail Mix (**160 calories, 10 g fat**)

✔ 1 oz (⅙ can) Planters Honey Roasted Peanuts (**160 calories, 13 g fat**)

✔ 1 oz (⅙ can) Planters Cocktail Peanuts (**170 calories, 1 g sugars**)

✔ ¼ cup Archer Farms Deluxe Roasted Mixed Nuts (**170 calories**)

Choose Your Mini Chocolate

Luckily it's easy to get your chocolate in small bites. See how many calories are in 1 piece of your favorite mini chocolate.

Hershey's Nugget Special Dark with Almonds	50
Reese's Peanut Butter Cups Miniature	44
Hershey's Miniature	42
Kit Kat Miniature Wafer	42
Hershey's Bliss Dark Chocolate	35
Hershey's Milk Chocolate with Almonds Kiss	23
Hershey's Special Dark Kiss	21

Appetizers and Snacks
CHEESE

✖ STOP EATING	✔ START EATING

🛒 Packaged

✖ 2 oz sliced provolone (199 calories, 15 g fat)

✖ 1-inch cube (1 oz) Cabot Seriously Sharp Cheddar (110 calories, 7 g protein)

✖ ¼ cup shredded 4-cheese Mexican blend (110 calories, 9 g fat)

✔ 1 Mini Babybel Light

KICK START

50 calories
3 g fat

✔ 1-inch cube (1 oz) Cabot Sharp Light Cheddar

KICK START

70 calories
8 g protein

✔ ¼ cup Kraft Shredded Reduced Fat Mild Cheddar

STEADY LOSS

80 calories
6 g fat

✔ 2 slices (1¼ oz) Sargento Thin Sliced Reduced Fat Provolone

STEADY LOSS

100 calories
7 g fat

Other Good Choices

✓ 1 Mini Babybel Original **(70 calories, 6 g fat)**

✓ ¼ cup Sargento Shredded Reduced Fat 4 Cheese Mexican **(80 calories, 6 g fat)**

✓ 2 slices (1¼ oz) Sargento Thin Sliced Reduced Fat Provolone **(100 calories, 6 g fat)**

✖ STOP EATING | ✔ START EATING

✘ *Restaurant*

✖ Half order Chili's Crispy Cheddar Bits (675 calories, 60 g fat)

✖ Cosi Brie & Fruit (500 calories)

✖ Create a Sampler portion Olive Garden Fried Mozzarella (420 calories, 24.5 g fat)

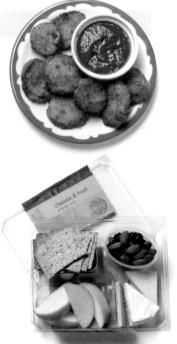

✔ 2 pieces (about ¼ order) Ruby Tuesday Fried Mozzarella with 2 Tbsp Tomato Basil Sauce

150 calories
9 g fat

MAINTAIN

✔ ½ Starbucks Cheese & Fruit Bistro Box

240 calories

MAINTAIN

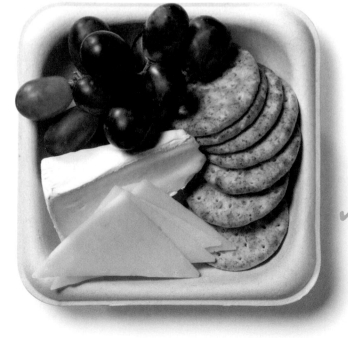

✔ Au Bon Pain Brie, Cheddar & Fruit with Crackers Petit Plate

310 calories

MAINTAIN

Chapter 15
DESERTS

What's life without dessert? I've never been an eat-dessert-every-night person, but I need room for something sweet in my daily diet, and our readers (and testers) have made it very clear that they do, too. So I strove to pick delicious options that offer good nutrition (yes, these desserts exist) or at least cut the obvious, over-the-top calories to take the sin out of sinfully sweet.

The magic word for dessert is *fruit*. It's elegant and satisfying by itself, or sometimes dusted with powdered sugar, or even topped with a small dollop of whipped cream. You get fiber, vitamins, and not many calories. Layer it with plain 0% Greek yogurt and a handful of nuts or granola, and you also add filling protein and tummy-trimming MUFAs. You can't go wrong. For a change of pace, buy frozen fruit. Freezing brings out the natural sugars in fruit, so they taste even sweeter. Try a frozen fruit salad of grapes, berries, pineapple, peach slices, mango, or whatever else you like. Or toss them in a blender or food processor to make an all-natural smoothie, sorbet, or frozen fruit pop. (See the "Fruit Swaps" chart on page 59 for calorie comparisons.) If you don't have time to make your own, I've recommended some frozen fruit bars and sorbets. Look for ones that don't add sugar or cream.

What about ice cream and its many relatives—frozen yogurt, gelato, and others? Of course, watching portion size is a given because of the calories from fat and sugar. But frozen dairy desserts do have an upside because many brands deliver a fair amount of calcium and some protein. You can look for products that cut out fat, sugar, or both, but you might have to try a few different brands to pick ones that are worth the swap tastewise. I found a few I like.

Puddings, custards, and mousses call for some of the same swaps as ice cream—you can drop the calories by getting rid of the fat, sugar, or both. You might want to make your own from a boxed mix. Or buy the ready-made cups because they're really easy, convenient, and in a just-right ½-cup portion size. Most restaurant servings are much bigger and richer (shorthand for more calories and fat) than what you'd have at home.

Calories in baked desserts such as cookies, cakes, brownies, and pies add up quickly because they contain not only fat and sugar but also flour. Every tablespoon of flour has nearly 30 calories, and an average cookie, for example, could contain several tablespoons; a piece of cake has even more. You can look for brands that have less sugar or fat, but the swap won't save you many calories and they usually don't taste as good. I'd rather choose a small cookie, cake pop, brownie bite, or minitart than try to be happy with a mediocre skinny product. (There are some exceptions, of course. I love how Skinny Cow Vanilla Ice Cream Sandwiches taste, and so did many of our testers!)

If you must have pastry or cake, you'll be surprised to know that we've selected some packaged goods (like Little Debbie's or Duncan Hines brownies) to help with portion control. You'll see, though, that our recommendations don't always follow what the package says. A serving of Oreos, for instance, is three cookies, but I suggest you stick to just two to keep the calorie count down.

STOP EATING	START EATING
• Premium ice creams with high amounts of fat	• Regular and lighter ice creams with less fat but great flavor
• Frozen fruit bars with cream or fatty coconut milk	• Frozen fruit bars with fruit plus juice and not much added sugar, preferably less than 5 grams
• Custards, puddings, crème brulee, and other restaurant desserts made with cream	• Milk-based puddings and custards made at home
• Full-size restaurant desserts	• One dessert to share at the table
• Oversized cakes, cookies, or brownies	• Mini desserts or baked desserts in one- or two-bite sizes, like a brownie bite
• Pies, especially double crust	• Fresh fruit

ICE CREAM AND OTHER FROZEN TREATS

✖ STOP EATING | ✔ START EATING

🛒 *Packaged*

✖ ½ cup Haagen-Dazs Dark Chocolate Chip Gelato (270 calories, 27 g sugars)

✖ Klondike Original Bar (250 calories, 8% calcium)

✖ Good Humor Vanilla King Cone (230 calories, 11 g fat)

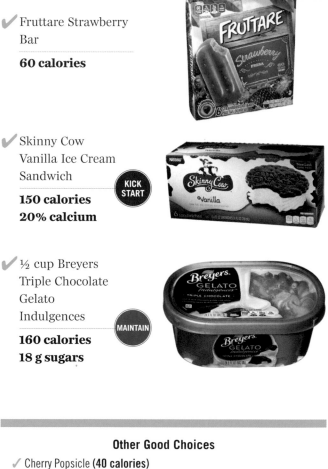

✔ Fruttare Strawberry Bar

60 calories

✔ Skinny Cow Vanilla Ice Cream Sandwich

KICK START

150 calories
20% calcium

✔ ½ cup Breyers Triple Chocolate Gelato Indulgences

MAINTAIN

160 calories
18 g sugars

Other Good Choices

✓ Cherry Popsicle **(40 calories)**

✓ Fruit Bar, No Sugar Added, any flavor **(60 calories)**

✓ Skinny Cow Chocolate Truffle Ice Cream Bar **(100 calories)**

✓ ½ cup Breyers Natural Vanilla **(130 calories, 14 g sugars)**

✓ ½ cup Haagen-Dazs Mango Sorbet **(150 calories, 10% vitamin C)**

✓ Klondike No Sugar Added Crunch Bar **(170 calories)**

✖ STOP EATING | ✔ START EATING

🍴 *Restaurant*

✖ Applebee's Chocolate Chip Cookie Sundae (1400 calories, 57 g fat)

✖ IHOP regular Ice Cream Sundae with Strawberry Topping (380 calories, 33 g sugars)

✖ McDonald's Hot Caramel Sundae (340 calories, 43 g sugars)

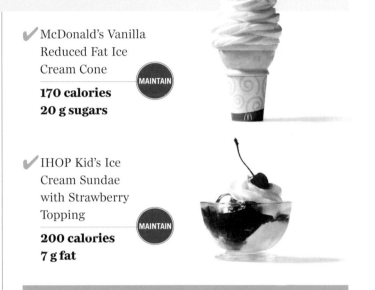

✔ McDonald's Vanilla Reduced Fat Ice Cream Cone

MAINTAIN

**170 calories
20 g sugars**

✔ IHOP Kid's Ice Cream Sundae with Strawberry Topping

MAINTAIN

**200 calories
7 g fat**

Other Good Choice

✓ ½ cup no-sugar-added 16 Handles Strawberry Fields yogurt **(72 calories, 8 g sugar)**

Desserts
COOKIES

<table>
<tr><td>

⊗ STOP EATING

</td><td>

✓ START EATING

</td></tr>
</table>

⊗ STOP EATING	✓ START EATING

🛒 *Packaged*

✖ 3 Nabisco Chips Ahoy! Original cookies (160 calories, 8 g fat)	✓ 2 Nabisco Ginger Snaps — **KICK START** — **60 calories**
✖ 1 bake-at-home Pillsbury Big Deluxe Oatmeal Raisin cookie (150 calories, 15 g sugars)	
✖ 8 Nabisco Nilla Wafers (140 calories)	✓ 2 Nabisco Oreos — **KICK START** — **106 calories** **4.5 g fat**

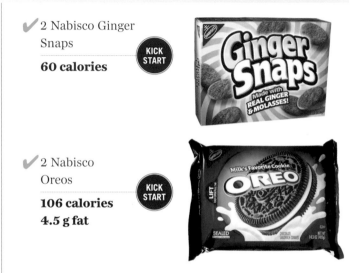

Other Good Choices

✓ 2 Nabisco Nilla Wafers (**35 calories**)

✓ 8 Miss Meringue Chocolate Mini Meringues (**68 calories**)

✓ 2 Trader Joe's Soft Bite Mini Almond Biscotti (**86 calories**)

✓ Weight Watchers Oatmeal Raisin Cookie (**90 calories, 2.5 g fat**)

✓ 1 Nonni's Originali Biscotti (**90 calories**)

✓ 3 Keebler Fudge Shoppe Cheesecake Middles Original Graham cookies (**130 calories**)

❌ STOP EATING | ✅ START EATING

❌ 1 Cosi Chocolate Chunk Cookie (448 calories, 40 g sugars)

❌ 1 Panera Oatmeal Raisin Cookie (400 calories, 32 g sugars)

❌ 1 Einstein Bros. Bagels Chocolate Chunk Cookie (390 calories, 31 g sugars)

✔ 1 Panera Petite Chocolate Chipper

100 calories
8 g sugars

MAINTAIN

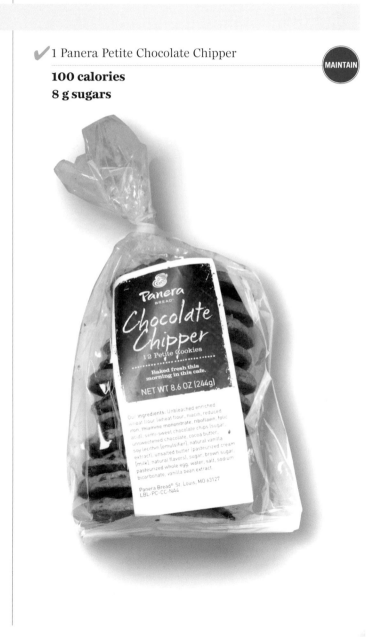

Desserts
CAKES, BROWNIES, AND BARS

❌ STOP EATING	✅ START EATING

🛒 *Packaged*

❌ ¼ Sara Lee Original Cream Strawberry Cheesecake (330 calories, 35 g sugars)

❌ Sara Lee Brownie Chocolate Chip Cake (⅐ package) (220 calories, 20 g sugars)

❌ 2-inch square brownie made from Ghirardelli Double Chocolate Brownie Mix (180 calories, 18 g sugars)

❌ 2½-inch square brownie made from Pillsbury Chocolate Fudge Brownie Mix (160 calories, 16 g sugars)

Other Good Choices

✓ 1 pouch (⅐ package) Special K Divine Fudge Brownies **(80 calories, 6 g sugars)**

✓ Weight Watchers Chocolate Creme Cake **(90 calories)**

✓ 1 pouch Entenmann'sLittle Bites Crumb Cakes **(230 calories, 11 g fat)**

✓ 1 pouch (⅐ package) Kellogg's Special K Blondie Mini Brownies   **KICK START**

100 calories
7 g sugars

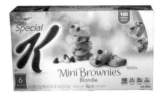

✓ 2 x 2½-inch brownie made from No Pudge! Original Fudge Brownie mix   **STEADY LOSS**

110 calories
0 g fat

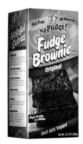

✓ 2½-inch square made from Duncan Hines Dark Chocolate Fudge Brownie mix   **MAINTAIN**

140 calories
15 g sugars

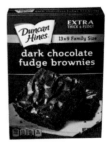

✓ 1 (1/10 box) Little Debbie Chocolate Chip Cake   **MAINTAIN**

150 calories
7 g fat

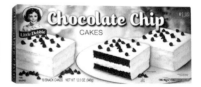

❌ STOP EATING | ✅ START EATING

❌ Applebee's Butter Pecan Blondie (1180 calories, 62 g fat)

❌ Denny's Hot Fudge Brownie a la Mode (830 calories, 95 g sugars)

❌ Einstein Bros. Bagels Chocolate Chip Coffee Cake (830 calories, 63 g sugars)

❌ Ruby Tuesday New York Cheesecake (758 calories, 60 g fat)

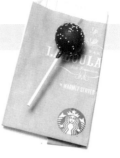

✅ Starbucks Chocolate Cake Pop

KICK START

140 calories
7 g fat

✅ 1 Maggiano's Chocolate Zuccotto Bite

KICK START

140 calories
14 g sugars

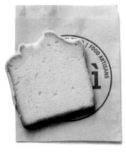

✅ ½ slice Cosi Lemon Pound Cake

MAINTAIN

235 calories
20.5 g sugars

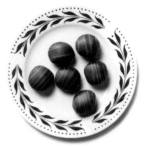

✅ Cosi Blondie Brownie

MAINTAIN

454 calories
34 g fat

Other Good Choices

✓ 1 order Au Bon Pain Brownie Bites (**160 calories, 15 g sugars**)

✓ Panera Cinnamon Crumb Coffee Cake (**220 calories, 14 g sugars**)

✓ Jersey Mike's Chocolate Brownie (**470 calories, 58 g sugars**)

Desserts
PIES AND TARTS

❌ **STOP EATING**	✅ **START EATING**

🏠 *Homemade*

❌ 1 slice (⅙ pie) double-crusted blueberry pie made from 2 Oronoque Orchards Deep Dish Pie Crusts and 1 can Comstock Blueberry Pie Filling (450 calories, 18 g fat)

✔ 1 slice (⅙ pie) blueberry pie made from 1 Oronoque Orchards Deep Dish Pie Crust and 1 can Comstock Blueberry Pie Filling

280 calories
9 g fat

MAINTAIN

✖ STOP EATING | ✔ START EATING

🛒 *Packaged*

✖ 1 slice (⅙ pie) Sara Lee Oven Fresh Blueberry Pie (350 calories, 16 g fat)

✖ ½ Marie Callender's frozen Key Lime Mini Pie (350 calories, 36 g sugars)

✖ ⅛ Mrs. Smith's Classic Apple Pie (340 calories, 17 g fat)

✔ ¼ Marie Callender's frozen Small Apple Pie

STEADY LOSS

170 calories
9 g sugars

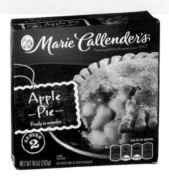

Other Good Choices

✔ ⅛ Sara Lee Oven Fresh Blueberry Pie (**262 calories, 15 g sugars**)

✔ ⅛ Sara Lee Pumpkin Pie (**270 calories, 32 g sugar**)

🍴 *Restaurant*

✖ 1 slice Marie Callender's restaurant Cherry Pie (600 calories, 39 g fat)

✖ Red Lobster Key Lime Pie (580 calories, 22 g fat)

✖ Burger King Dutch Apple Pie (340 calories, 23 g sugars)

✔ McDonald's Baked Hot Apple Pie

MAINTAIN

250 calories
4 g fiber

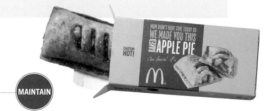

Other Good Choics

✔ KFC Apple Turnover (**230 calories, 10 g fat**)

Desserts
PUDDINGS AND CUSTARDS

✖ STOP EATING | ✔ START EATING

🛒 *Packaged*

✖ ½ cup prepared Jell-O Instant Pudding and Pie Filling with fat-free milk (130 calories, 18 g sugars)

✖ ½ cup Kozy Shack Original Rice Pudding (120 calories, 14 g sugars)

✖ Snack Pack Tapioca Pudding (110 calories, 13 g sugars)

✔ ½ cup prepared Royal Instant Sugar Free Reduced Calorie Pudding with fat-free milk

KICK START

80 calories

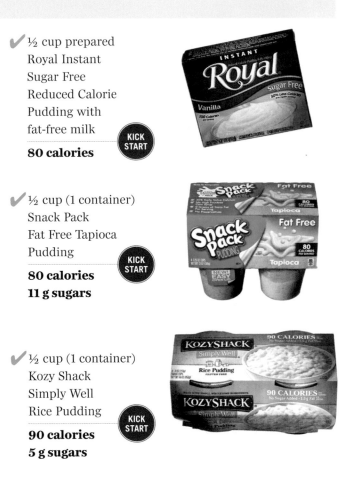

✔ ½ cup (1 container) Snack Pack Fat Free Tapioca Pudding

KICK START

80 calories
11 g sugars

✔ ½ cup (1 container) Kozy Shack Simply Well Rice Pudding

KICK START

90 calories
5 g sugars

✖ STOP EATING | ## ✔ START EATING

✗ *Restaurant*

✖ Olive Garden Black
Tie Mousse Cake
(770 calories, 52 g fat)

✖ Ruby Tuesday Tiramisu
(555 calories,
30 g fat)

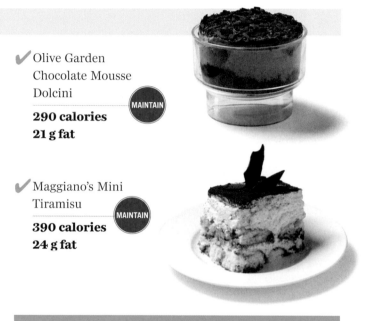

✔ Olive Garden
Chocolate Mousse
Dolcini

MAINTAIN

**290 calories
21 g fat**

✔ Maggiano's Mini
Tiramisu

MAINTAIN

**390 calories
24 g fat**

Other Good Choices

✓ ½ cup Souplantation Sugar-Free Chocolate Mousse (**40 calories,
1 g sugars**)

✓ Olive Garden Amaretto Tiramisu Dolcini (**220 calories, 17 g fat**)

✓ Maggiano's Mini Crème Brulee (**260 calories, 18 g fat**)

FRUIT-BASED DESSERTS

✖ STOP EATING | ✓ START EATING

✖ Blueberry crumble made with 1 cup blueberries, baked with a topping of 2 Tbsp granola, 1 Tbsp butter, 1 Tbsp walnuts, and 2 tsp sugar (314 calories)

✓ Blueberry crumble made with 1 cup blueberries, and a topping of 1 Tbsp each oats and sliced almonds, ½ tsp butter, 1 tsp sugar, and ¼ tsp cinnamon

188 calories

STEADY LOSS

HOW TO MAKE IT

Place 1 cup blueberries in a 1½-cup ovenproof ramekin. Crumble together 1 Tbsp each oats and sliced almonds, ½ tsp butter, 1 tsp sugar, and ¼ tsp cinnamon in a small bowl. Sprinkle over the blueberries. Bake at 350°F until bubbly and lightly browned, about 20 minutes. (Makes 1 serving)

❌ STOP EATING | ✅ START EATING

🍴 *Restaurant*

❌ Longhorn Steakhouse Caramel Apple Goldrush (1640 calories, 71 g fat)

✔ Cosi Non-Fat Greek Yogurt Parfait

300 calories
0 g fat

MAINTAIN

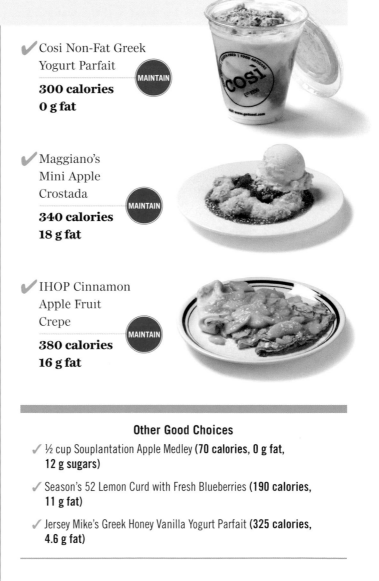

✔ Maggiano's Mini Apple Crostada

340 calories
18 g fat

MAINTAIN

✔ IHOP Cinnamon Apple Fruit Crepe

380 calories
16 g fat

MAINTAIN

Other Good Choices

✓ ½ cup Souplantation Apple Medley (**70 calories, 0 g fat, 12 g sugars**)

✓ Season's 52 Lemon Curd with Fresh Blueberries (**190 calories, 11 g fat**)

✓ Jersey Mike's Greek Honey Vanilla Yogurt Parfait (**325 calories, 4.6 g fat**)

Chapter 16
DRINKS

As a kid, I refused to drink water. Even when I was dying of thirst, I just found it too plain and boring. Then, after college, I read an interview with an athlete who said that drinking water was her secret to peak performance. So I forced myself to drink my eight glasses a day. Now I drink almost nothing else—just a morning cup of tea and then fresh cold water the rest of the day, sometimes flavored with lemon, ginger, or other fruits and herbs.

The thing to remember with drinks is that most are not very filling. So any drinks with calories take away from your food calories and may leave you feeling less satisfied. But of course some occasions do call for a drink: an ice-cold beer at a ball game, a glass of lemonade after a day at the park with the girls, a cup of coffee after dinner at our favorite Italian restaurant. The good news is you don't need to limit yourself to calorie-free drinks for the rest of your life. You just need to make smart choices on the rare occasions when you indulge in your favorite beverage. In this chapter, I'm sharing with you a variety of drinks, from wine and other alcoholic beverages to coffee and tea drinks, milks, and juices. Each has its own rules.

Did you know that wines from countries with warmer climates, such as Australia and Chile, have more calories per sip than wines from the cooler European countries? The warm weather grapes are higher in sugar, and more sugar on the vine means more alcohol in the wine. Red wines and white wines can have similar calories because calories depend more on sugar and alcohol than on color. But sparkling wines like champagne and prosecco are a bit lower calorie, so bring them on. You can drop calories just by switching to a wine with less alcohol, listed as ABV (alcohol by volume). That same rule can apply to beer. A lot of restaurants and brew pubs list the percentage of alcohol in the beers they carry. If you don't see it on the menu, the bartender may know. Most beers, by the way, are about the same number of calories—light beers are generally around 100 calories per 12-ounce bottle, regular beers around 150 calories.

Traditional spirits—vodka, gin, bourbon, whiskey, and others—have about the same number of calories per ounce. With cocktails, the best way to drop calories is to swap mixers. Instead of sweet juices or nectars, choose a drink made with seltzer or a squeeze of lemon or lime juice. Try your rum and coke or gin and tonic with diet soda. And unless a restaurant serves one of the skinny brands, there's no way to decrease the calories in frozen drinks like margaritas, daiquiris, and piña coladas except to drink less. Downsizing your drink is, of course, always a good option.

The government's Dietary Guidelines and health experts recommend that adults have three daily servings of dairy products to get the calcium needed for healthy bones. I love milk and cheese, but the calories can really add up if I choose full-fat versions. I personally could never get used to the taste of plain fat-free milk, but in a latte or cappuccino, where the milk foams up really well, I don't notice the difference. Depending on the size, a coffee drink can have one or even two cups of milk. As I've gotten older, I've developed some lactose intolerance, so I started using calcium-fortified soy or almond milk in my lattes instead. Both are generally easy to find at the market and in your local café. (Of course, you can also get calcium from other types of food, including leafy greens.)

In drinks like iced tea, lemonade, juice drinks, and soft drinks, every single calorie comes from sugar. So unless they're unsweetened, I have them only once in a while as a treat. Still, I found a few products to recommend. I personally don't like artificial sweeteners, but calorie-free teas and sodas can be a good option occasionally.

Be wary of drinks with a health halo. Fruit juices are especially deceptive. They do include more vitamins and other nutrients than sodas, but even those advertised as containing 100% fresh fruit have more calories and more sugar (and less fiber) than the fruit they're made from. And you'll notice that I did not include enhanced waters and energy drinks. While they may include some vitamins or electrolytes, most of them are really just sugar water. Even coconut water, the clear liquid from the middle of the coconut, doesn't offer much in the way of nutrition (though it is, at least, lower in calories than fatty coconut milk).

STOP EATING	START EATING
• Wines and beers with higher alcohol content	• Wines (often European) and beers with lower alcohol content
• Frozen cocktails and drinks made with supersweet mixers like margarita mix, other bottled mixes, or fruit nectar	• A splash of fruit juice mixed with seltzer, just seltzer by itself, or light mixers
• Coffee, tea, chai, and hot cocoa made with whole milk or full-fat nondairy milks	• Coffee, tea, chai, and hot cocoa (light or sugar-free) made with fat-free milk and lower-fat nondairy milks
• Sugar-sweetened iced teas, lemonades, and soft drinks	• Unsweetened, lightly sweetened, or calorie-free cold beverages

Drinks
WINE AND BEER

❌ STOP DRINKING | ## ✅ START DRINKING

🛒 *Packaged*

❌ 12-oz bottle Sam Adams Double Bock (330 calories)

❌ 12-oz bottle Angry Orchard Hard Cider (200 calories)

❌ 6 oz Gewurztraminer (200 calories)

❌ 6 oz Australian or Chilean red wine (ABV 13.5–16%) (180 calories)

✓ 12-oz bottle Dos Equis XX
145 calories STEADY LOSS

✓ 6 oz European red wine (ABV 11–13.5%)
155 calories STEADY LOSS

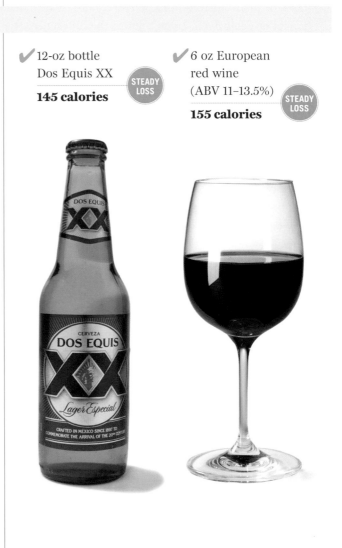

Other Good Choices

✓ 12-oz bottle O'Doul's (alcohol-free) **(70 calories)**

✓ 12-oz bottle Amstel Light **(95 calories)**

✓ 12-oz bottle Coors Light **(102 calories)**

✓ 12-oz bottle Bud Light **(110 calories)**

✓ 6 oz Pinot Grigio **(125 calories)**

✓ 6 oz champagne **(128 calories)**

✓ 2-oz bottle Woodpecker Premium Cider **(150 calories)**

✓ 12-oz bottle Michelob **(155 calories)**

✓ START DRINKING

🛒 *Packaged*

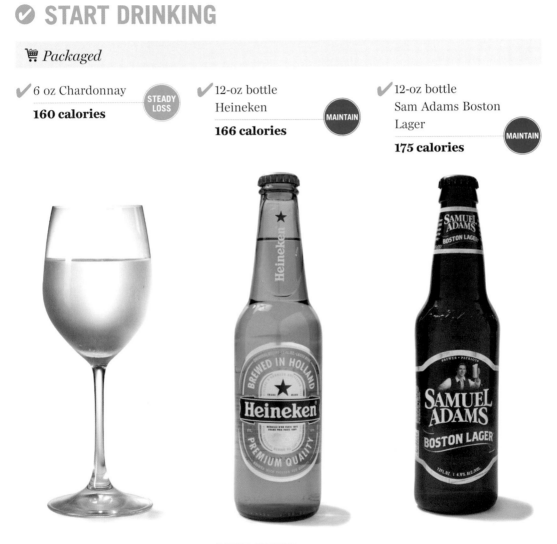

✓ 6 oz Chardonnay

160 calories

STEADY LOSS

✓ 12-oz bottle Heineken

166 calories

MAINTAIN

✓ 12-oz bottle Sam Adams Boston Lager

175 calories

MAINTAIN

SUPER SWITCH
Switch to a 12-oz bottle of Heineken Light and drop another 67 calories

Drinks
COCKTAILS

❌ STOP DRINKING | ✅ START DRINKING

🍴 *Restaurant*

❌ 7 oz chocolate martini
(438 calories)

❌ 6 oz piña colada
(378 calories)

❌ Olive Garden Margarita
(340 calories)

❌ Longhorn Steakhouse
White Peach Sangria
(230 calories)

✔ ½ cup Master of Mixes Lite Margarita Mixer,
1½ oz tequila

KICK START

106 calories

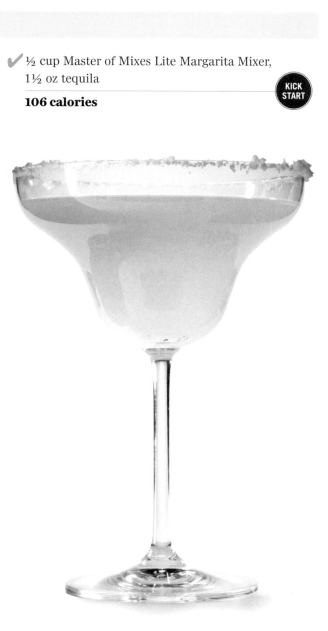

✓ START DRINKING

✓ Mimosa with 4 oz champagne, and 2 oz orange juice

KICK START

114 calories

✓ Longhorn Steakhouse Skinny Black Raspberry Sangria

STEADY LOSS

160 calories

✓ Cosmopolitan 4 oz

MAINTAIN

200 calories

✓ Olive Garden Mojito

MAINTAIN

210 calories

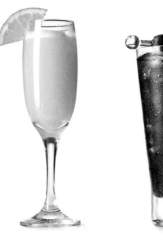

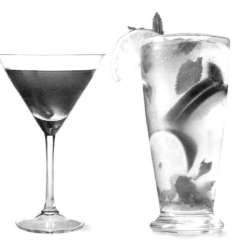

Other Good Choices

✓ Carrabba's Skinny Rita **(109 calories)**

✓ Rum and Coke **(185 calories)**

✓ Bloody Mary **(189 calories)**

✓ Screwdriver **(190 calories)**

✓ ½ cup Margaritaville Margarita Mix, 1½ oz tequila **(206 calories)**

✓ 4 oz classic martini

MAINTAIN

256 calories

SUPER SWITCH
Switch to a 3 oz green apple martini and drop another 108 calories

Drinks
COFFEE

✖ STOP DRINKING	✔ START DRINKING

✗ *Restaurant*

✖ Small (12 oz) McDonald's Caramel Frappe (440 calories, 57 g sugars)

✖ Small (16 oz) Dunkin' Donuts Vanilla Bean Coolatta (420 calories, 87 g sugars)

✔ 12 oz coffee with 2 Tbsp (1 oz) whole milk

17 calories

KICK START

SUPER SWITCH
Switch to 12 oz coffee with fat-free milk and drop an additional 7 calories

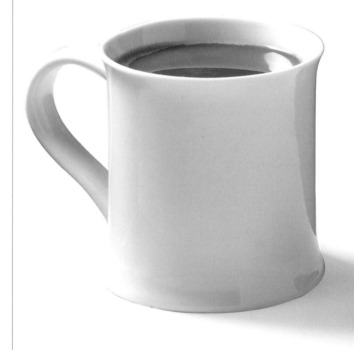

Choose Your Milk or Creamer

Coffee itself has no calories. It's the milk or creamer and sugar that you add that's the problem. See how many calories are in common whiteners, per 2 tablespoons.

Coffee-mate Original	40
Half-and-half	39
Fat-free half-and-half	17
Whole milk	17
2% milk	16
Skim Plus milk	14
Low-fat (1% fat) milk	13
Fat-free milk	10
Silk Original Almond Milk	8
Silk Light Original Soymilk	8

✕ STOP DRINKING | ✓ START DRINKING

✗ Restaurant

✗ Grande (16 oz) Starbucks Caramel Flan Latte made with whole milk, no whipped cream (280 calories, 10 g fat)

✓ Tall (12 oz) Starbucks nonfat cappuccino

KICK START

60 calories

✓ Small (12 oz) Caribou Latte with fat-free milk

KICK START

90 calories
12 g sugars

✓ Tall (12 oz) Starbucks Caramel Frappuccino Light

STEADY LOSS

100 calories
0 g fat

✓ Dunkin' Donuts Medium (16 oz) Latte Lite

STEADY LOSS

120 calories

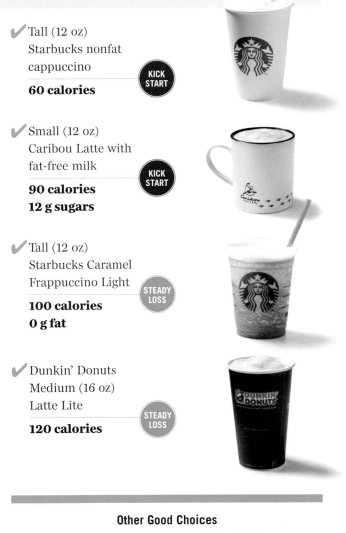

Other Good Choices

✓ 12 oz coffee with fat-free half-and-half **(17 calories)**

✓ Tall (12 oz) Starbucks cappuccino with 2% milk **(90 calories)**

✓ Grande (16 oz) Starbucks Flavored Skinny Latte **(120 calories)**

❌ STOP DRINKING | ✅ START DRINKING

🏠 *Homemade*

❌ 2 Tbsp Pacific Chai Spice Chai Latte in ¾ cup (6 oz) hot water (90 calories)

✔ Tea with 2 Tbsp (1 oz) whole milk and chai spices

19 calories

KICK START

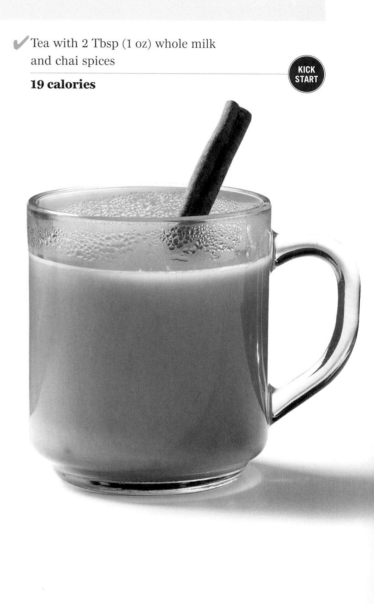

⊗ STOP DRINKING | ⊘ START DRINKING

🛒 *Packaged*

✖ 16-oz bottle Snapple
Half 'n Half
(210 calories,
50 g sugars)

✖ 16-oz bottle Arizona
Iced Tea with Lemon
Flavor (180 calories,
48 g sugars)

✔ 16-oz can Steaz Zero
Calorie Iced Green
Tea Half & Half

KICK START

0 calories
0 g sugars

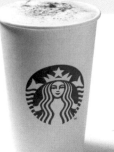

✔ 20-oz bottle Lipton
Lemon Iced Tea

MAINTAIN

120 calories
31 g sugars

Other Good Choices

✓ 16-oz bottle Honest T Mango White
Tea **(70 calories, 18 g sugars)**

✓ 16-oz can Steaz Half and Half
Iced Green Tea **(80 calories,
18 g sugars)**

✓ 16-oz bottle Snapple Green Tea
(120 calories, 30 g sugars)

✓ 14-oz bottle Tazo Giant Peach Iced
Tea **(150 calories, 36 g sugars)**

✔ 16-oz bottle Snapple
Green Tea

MAINTAIN

120 calories
30 g sugars

🍴 *Restaurant*

✖ Tall (12 oz) Starbucks
Iced Teavana Green Tea
Latte (210 calories)

✔ Tall (12 oz)
Starbucks Teavana
Oprah Cinnamon
Chai Tea Latte with
nonfat milk

MAINTAIN

130 calories

Drinks
MILK

❌ STOP DRINKING | ✅ START DRINKING

🛒 *Packaged*

❌ 1 cup (8 oz) whole milk
(149 calories, 8 g fat)

❌ 1 cup (8 oz) Silk Very Vanilla
Soymilk (130 calories,
3.5 g fat)

✅ 1 cup (8 oz) fat-free milk

83 calories
0 g fat

KICK
START

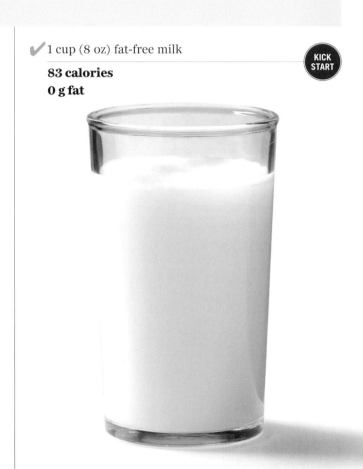

Choose Your Milk

Does it really make a difference to go skim? See how many calories and how much fat are in
a cup of different types of milk.

Whole milk.....................................**149 calories, 8 g fat**	Low fat (1% milk) ....**102 calories, 2.5 g fat**	
Reduced fat (2% milk)...............**122 calories, 5 g fat**	Fat-free milk ....**83 calories, 0 g fat**	
Skim Plus milk ....**110 calories, 0 g fat**		

✅ START DRINKING

🛒 *Packaged*

✔️ 1 cup (8 oz) Silk Original
Almond Milk

KICK START

60 calories
45% calcium

SUPER SWITCH
Switch to Silk Original
Unsweetened Almond Milk
and drop another 30 calories

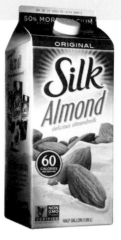

Other Good Choices

✓ 1 cup (8 oz) Almond Breeze
Original Unsweetened
Almond Milk **(30 calories)**

✓ 1 cup (8 oz) Silk
Unsweetened Coconut Milk
(45 calories, 4 g fat)

✓ 1 cup (8 oz) Silk Light
Original Soymilk
(60 calories, 3 g sugars)

✔️ 1 cup (8 oz) Coconut
Dream Unsweetened
Coconut Milk

KICK START

60 calories
5 g fat

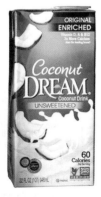

✔️ 1 cup (8 oz) Westsoy
Organic Unsweetened
Soymilk

KICK START

90 calories
4.5 g fat

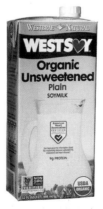

Drinks
FRUIT JUICES AND SODAS

⊗ STOP DRINKING | ✓ START DRINKING

🛒 _Packaged_

✖ 12-oz can Coca-Cola
(150 calories, 39 g
sugars)

✖ 1 cup orange juice
(120 calories)

✖ 12-oz bottle IZZE
Sparkling Clementine
(120 calories,
27 g sugars)

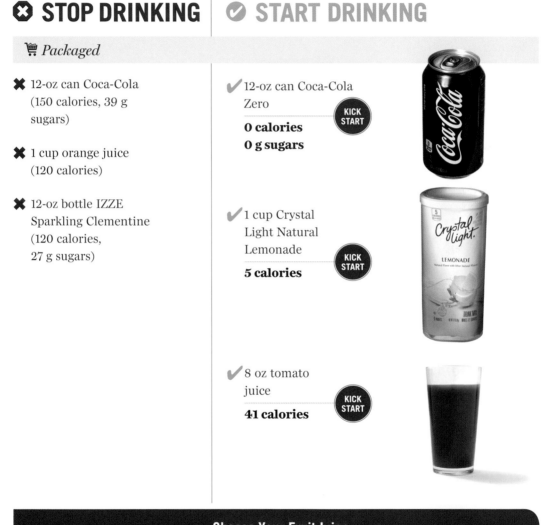

✓ 12-oz can Coca-Cola
Zero
KICK START
0 calories
0 g sugars

✓ 1 cup Crystal
Light Natural
Lemonade
KICK START
5 calories

✓ 8 oz tomato
juice
KICK START
41 calories

Choose Your Fruit Juice

Consider how many calories and grams of sugars are in common fruit juices, per 8 ounces.

Grape juice........................ **152 calories, 36 g sugars**		Grapefruit juice................... **96 calories, 23 g sugars**
Cranberry juice.................. **137 calories, 30 g sugars**		Cranberry juice, light............ **50 calories, 11 g sugars**
Orange juice...................... **122 calories, 21 g sugars**		Tomato juice.......................... **41 calories, 9 g sugars**
Apple juice .... **114 calories, 24 g sugars**		

⊘ START DRINKING

🛒 *Packaged*

✔ 1 cup Trop50
No Pulp Calcium +
Vitamin D

**KICK
START**

50 calories
35% calcium

✔ 12-oz bottle Gus
Extra Dry
Ginger Ale

**STEADY
LOSS**

90 calories

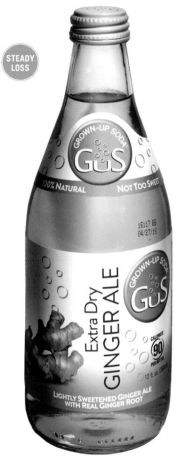

Other Good Choice

✓ 12-oz bottle IZZE Esque Sparkling Limon (**50 calories,
11 g sugars**)

NOTES

1. National Cancer Institute Applied Research: Cancer Control and Population Sciences, Table 3, http://appliedresearch.cancer.gov/diet/foodsources/food_groups/table3.html.

2. D. Mozaffarian et al., "Trans Fatty Acids and Cardiovascular Disease," *New England Journal of Medicine* 354 (April 13, 2006): 1601–13, www.nejm.org/doi/full/10.1056/NEJMra054035.

3. M. Wang et al., "Association between Sugar-Sweetened Beverages and Type 2 Diabetes: A Meta-Analysis," *Journal of Diabetes Investigation* 6, no. 3 (May 2015): 360–66, www.ncbi.nlm.nih.gov/pubmed/25969723.

4. J. Ma et al., "Sugar-Sweetened Beverage, Diet Soda, and Fatty Liver Disease in the Framingham Heart Study Cohorts," *Journal of Hepatology*, May 29, 2015, www.ncbi.nlm.nih.gov/pubmed/26055949.

5. U.S. Department of Agriculture and U.S. Department of Health and Human Services, *Dietary Guidelines for Americans, 2010*, 7th ed. (Washington, DC: U.S. Government Printing Office, 2010).

6. B. Wansink and J. Kim, "Bad Popcorn in Big Buckets: Portion Size Can Influence Intake as Much as Taste," *Journal of Nutrition Education and Behavior* 37, no. 5 (September–October 2005): 242–45.

7. N. Diliberti, "Increased Portion Size Leads to Increased Energy Intake in a Restaurant Meal," *Obesity Research* 12, no. 3 (March 2004): 562–68, www.ncbi.nlm.nih.gov/pubmed/15044675.

8. J. E. Flood, L. S. Roe, and B. J. Rolls, "The Effect of Increased Beverage Portion Size on Energy Intake at a Meal," *Journal of the American Dietetic Association* 106, no. 12 (December 2006): 1984–90, www.ncbi.nlm.nih.gov/pubmed/17126628.

9. Lisa R. Young and Marion Nestle, "Expanding Portion Sizes in the US Marketplace: Implications for Nutrition Counseling," *Journal of the American Dietetic Association* 103, no. 2 (February 2003): 231–34, http://portionteller.com/pdf/portsize.pdf.

10. G. O'Loughlin et al., "Using a Wearable Camera to Increase the Accuracy of Dietary Analysis," *American Journal of Preventive Medicine* 44, no. 3 (March 2013): 297–301, www.ncbi.nlm.nih.gov/pubmed/23415128.

11. "Beating Mindless Eating," Cornell University Food and Brand Lab, http://foodpsychology.cornell.edu/content/beating-mindless-eating.

12. M. Reicks et al., "Associations between Eating Occasion Characteristics and Age, Gender, Presence of Children and BMI among U.S. Adults," *Journal of the American College of Nutrition* 33, no. 4 (2014): 315–27, www.ncbi.nlm.nih.gov/pubmed/25140673.

13. E. Robinson, P. Aveyard, and S. A. Jebb, "Is Plate Clearing a Risk Factor for Obesity? A Cross-Sectional Study of Self-Reported Data in US Adults," *Obesity* (Silver Spring) 23, no. 2 (February 2015): 301–4, www.ncbi.nlm.nih.gov/pubmed/25521278.

14. M. Spence et al., "A Qualitative Study of Psychological, Social and Behavioral Barriers to Appropriate Food Portion Size Control," *International Journal of Behavioral Nutrition and Physical Activity* 10 (August 1, 2013): 92, www.ncbi.nlm.nih.gov/pubmed/23915381.

15. E. Robinson et al., "Eating Attentively: A Systematic Review and Meta-Analysis of the Effect of Food Intake Memory and Awareness on Eating," *American Journal of Clinical Nutrition* 97, no. 4 (April 2013): 728–42, www.ncbi.nlm.nih.gov/pubmed/23446890.

16. U.S. Department of Agriculture, www.choosemyplate.gov.

17. U.S. Department of Agriculture, Agricultural Research Service, "What We Eat in America," NHANES 2011–2012, individuals 2 years and over (excluding breast-fed children), day 1. www.ars.usda.gov/nea/bhnrc/fsrg, www.ars.usda.gov/SP2UserFiles/Place/80400530/pdf/1112/Table_53_RST_GEN_11.pdf.

18. U.S. Department of Agriculture, Economic Research Service, "Food-Away-from-Home," last updated October 29, 2014, www.ers.usda.gov/topics/food-choices-health/food-consumption-demand/food-away-from-home.aspx#nutrition.

19. G. B. Taksler and B. Elbel, "Calorie Labeling and Consumer Estimation of Calories Purchased," *International Journal of Behavioral Nutrition and Physical Activity* 11 (July 12, 2014): 91, www.ncbi.nlm.nih.gov/pubmed/25015547.

20. Josh Barro et al., "What 2,000 Calories Looks Like," *New York Times*, updated December 20, 2014, www.nytimes.com/interactive/2014/12/22/upshot/what-2000-calories-looks-like.html?_r=0&abt=0002&abg=1.

21. Jayne Hurley and Bonnie Liebman, "Extreme Eating 2015," *Nutrition Action Healthletter*, June 2015, www.cspinet.org/new/pdf/xtreme2015.pdf.

22. U.S. Food and Drug Administration, "Overview of FDA Labeling Requirements for Restaurants, Similar Retail Food Establishments and Vending Machines," last updated July 9, 2015, www.fda.gov/Food/IngredientsPackagingLabeling/LabelingNutrition/ucm248732.htm.

23. Chipotle, "Food with Integrity," www.chipotle.com/food-with-integrity.

24. Kevin Quealy, Amanda Cox, and Josh Katz, "At Chipotle, How Many Calories Do People Really Eat?" *New York Times*, February 17, 2015, www.nytimes.com/interactive/2015/02/17/upshot/what-do-people-actually-order-at-chipotle.html?abt=0002&abg=0&_r=1.

25. KIND, "Nice to Meet You, We're KIND," www.kindsnacks.com/about/#slide-three.

26. U.S. Food and Drug Administration, "KIND, LLC 3/17/15: Warning Letter," www.fda.gov/ICECI/EnforcementActions/WarningLetters/ucm440942.htm.

27. KIND, "A Note to Our KIND Community," April 14, 2015, www.kindsnacks.com/blog/post/a-note-to-our-kind-community-2/.

28. David Benton, "Portion Size: What We Know and What We Need to Know," *Critical Reviews in Food Science and Nutrition* 55, no. 7 (June 7, 2015): 988–1004, www.ncbi.nlm.nih.gov/pmc/articles/PMC4337741/.

29. B. Wansink and P. Chandon, "Can Low-Fat Nutrition Labels Lead to Obesity?" *Journal of Marketing Research* 43, no. 4 (November 2006): 605–17.

30. R. An, "Fast-Food and Full-Service Restaurant Consumption and Daily Energy and Nutrient Intakes in US Adults," *European Journal of Clinical Nutrition*, July 1, 2015, www.nature.com/ejcn/journal/vaop/ncurrent/full/ejcn2015104a.html.

31. K. Milton, "Hunter-Gatherer Diets—A Different Perspective," *American Journal of Clinical Nutrition* 71, no. 3 (March 2000): 665–67, http://ajcn.nutrition.org/content/71/3/665.full.

32. K. Kouda et al., "Metabolic Response to Short-Term 4-Day Energy Restriction in a Controlled Study," *Environmental Health and Preventive Medicine* 11, no. 2 (March 2006): 89–92, www.ncbi.nlm.nih.gov/pubmed/21432368.

33. C. E. O'Neil, T. A. Nicklas, and V. L. Fulgoni, "Nutrient Intake, Diet Quality, and Weight/Adiposity Parameters in Breakfast Patterns Compared with No Breakfast in Adults: National Health and Nutrition Examination Survey 2001-2008," *Journal of the Academy of Nutrition and Dietetics*, 114, no. S12 (December 2014): S27–43, www.ncbi.nlm.nih.gov/pubmed/25458992.

34. K. D. Hall et al., "Quantification of the Effect of Energy Imbalance on Bodyweight," *Lancet* 378, no. 9793 (August 27, 2011): 826–37, www.ncbi.nlm.nih.gov/pubmed/21872751.

35. "Mean intake of energy and mean contribution (kcal) of various U.S. foods among U.S. population, by age, NHANES 2005–2006," cited in the 2010 Dietary Guidelines Committee Report, http://www.cnpp.usda.gov/sites/default/files/dietary_guidelines_for_americans/2010DGACReport-camera-ready-Jan11-11.pdf

36. Kouda et al., "Metabolic Response to Short-Term 4-Day Energy Restriction," 89–92.

37. A. J. Hill, "The Psychology of Food Craving," *Proceedings of the Nutrition Society* 66, no. 2 (May 2007): 277–85, www.ncbi.nlm.nih.gov/pubmed/17466108.

38. National Weight Control Registry, http://www.nwcr.ws/research/.

39. R. M. Ryan and C. Frederick, "On Energy, Personality, and Health: Subjective Vitality as a Dynamic Reflection of Well-Being," *Journal of Personality* 65, no. 3 (September 1997): 529–65, www.ncbi.nlm.nih.gov/pubmed/9327588.

40. M. L. Loureiro, S. T. Yen, and R. M. Nayga Jr., "The Effects of Nutritional Labels on Obesity," *Agricultural Economics* 43, no. 3 (May 2012): 333–42, http://onlinelibrary.wiley.com/doi/10.1111/j.1574-0862.2012.00586.x/abstract.

41. L. M. Nackers, K. M. Ross, and M. G. Perri, "The Association between Rate of Initial Weight Loss and Long-Term Success in Obesity Treatment: Does Slow and Steady Win the Race?" *International Journal of Behavioral Medicine* 17, no. 3 (September 2010): 161–67, www.ncbi.nlm.nih.gov/pubmed/20443094.

42. A. Astrup and S. Rossner, "Lessons from Obesity Management Programmes: Greater Initial Weight Loss Improves Long-Term Maintenance," *Obesity Reviews* 1, no. 1 (May 2000): 17–19, www.ncbi.nlm.nih.gov/pubmed/12119640.

43. E. J. Dhurandhar et al., "Predicting Adult Weight Change in the Real World: A Systematic Review and Meta-Analysis Accounting for Compensatory Changes in Energy Intake or Expenditure," *International Journal of Obesity* (London), October 17, 2014, www.ncbi.nlm.nih.gov/pubmed/25323965.

44. "Calories Burned in 30 Minutes for People of Three Different Weights," http://www.health.harvard.edu/diet-and-weight-loss/calories-burned-in-30-minutes-of-leisure-and-routine-activities (accessed July 20, 2015).

45. S. Hanson and A. Jones, "Is There Evidence That Walking Groups Have Health Benefits? A Systematic Review and Meta-Analysis," *British Journal of Sports Medicine* 49, no. 11 (June 2015): 710–15, www.ncbi.nlm.nih.gov/pubmed/25601182.

46. A. E. Field, "Dietary Fat and Weight Gain Among Women in the Nurses' Health Study," *Obesity* 15, no. 4 (April 2007): 967–76, http://onlinelibrary.wiley.com/doi/10.1038/oby.2007.616/full.

47. C. A. Grimes et al., "Dietary Salt Intake, Sugar-Sweetened Beverage Consumption, and Obesity Risk," *Pediatrics* 131, no. 1 (January 1, 2013): 14–21, http://pediatrics.aappublications.org/content/131/1/14.

48. V. S. Malik, M. B. Schulze, and F. B. Hu, "Intake of Sugar-Sweetened Beverages and Weight Gain: A Systematic Review," *American Journal of Clinical Nutrition* 84, no. 2 (August 2006): 274–88, www.ncbi.nlm.nih.gov/pmc/articles/PMC3210834/.

49. A. R. Josse et al., "Increased Consumption of Dairy Foods and Protein during Diet- and Exercise-Induced Weight Loss Promotes Fat Mass Loss and Lean Mass Gain in Overweight and Obese Premenopausal Women," *Journal of Nutrition* 141, no. 9 (September 1, 2011): 1626–34, http://jn.nutrition.org/content/141/9/1626.short.

50. P. J. Weijs and R. R. Wolfe, "Exploration of the Protein Requirement during Weight Loss in Obese Older Adults," *Clinical Nutrition* (Edinburgh, Scotland), March 6, 2015, www.ncbi.nlm.nih.gov/pubmed/25788405.

51. D. H. Pesta and V. T. Samuel, "A High-Protein Diet for Reducing Body Fat: Mechanisms and Possible Caveats," *Nutrition & Metabolism* 11, no. 1 (November 19, 2014): 53, www.ncbi.nlm.nih.gov/pubmed/25489333.

52. A. Geliebter et al., "Effects of Oatmeal and Corn Flakes Cereal Breakfasts on Satiety, Gastric Emptying, Glucose, and Appetite-Related Hormones," *Annals of Nutrition & Metabolism* 66, nos. 2–3 (2015): 93–103, www.ncbi.nlm.nih.gov/pubmed/25612907.

53. S. Krishnan and J. A. Cooper, "Effect of Dietary Fatty Acid Composition on Substrate Utilization and Body Weight Maintenance in Humans," *European Journal of Nutrition* 53, no. 3 (April 2014): 691–710, www.ncbi.nlm.nih.gov/pubmed/24363161.

54. A. Due et al., "Comparison of 3 Ad Libitum Diets for Weight-Loss Maintenance, Risk of Cardiovascular Disease, and Diabetes: A 6-mo Randomized, Controlled Trial," *American Journal of Clinical Nutrition* 88, no. 5 (November 2008): 1232–41, www.ncbi.nlm.nih.gov/pubmed/18996857.

55. H. Wang et al., "Longitudinal Association between Dairy Consumption and Changes of Body Weight and Waist Circumference: The Framingham Heart Study," *International Journal of Obesity* (London) 38, no. 2 (February 2014): 299–305, www.ncbi.nlm.nih.gov/pubmed/23736371.

56. D. Canoy et al., "Plasma Ascorbic Acid Concentrations and Fat Distribution in 19,068 British Men and Women in the European Prospective Investigation into Cancer and Nutrition Norfolk Cohort Study," *American Journal of Clinical Nutrition* 82, no. 6 (December 2005): 1203–9, www.ncbi.nlm.nih.gov/pubmed/16332652.

57. K. Casazza et al., "Weighing the Evidence of Common Beliefs in Obesity Research," *Critical Reviews in Food Science and Nutrition* 55, no. 14 (December 6, 2015): 2014–53, www.ncbi.nlm.nih.gov/pubmed/24950157.

58. J. G. Thomas et al., "Weight-Loss Maintenance for 10 years in the National Weight Control Registry," *American Journal of Preventive Medicine* 46, no. 1 (2014): 17–23, www.ajpmonline.org/article/S0749-3797(13)00528-X/pdf.

59. M. Stead et al., "Why Are Some People More Successful at Lifestyle Change Than Others? Factors Associated with Successful Weight Loss in the BeWEL Randomised Controlled Trial of Adults at Risk of Colorectal Cancer," *International Journal of Behavioral Nutrition and Physical Activity* 12 (June 26, 2015): 87, www.ncbi.nlm.nih.gov/pubmed/26112014.

60. P. Ferrari et al., "Evaluation of Under- and Overreporting of Energy Intake in the 24-Hour Diet Recalls in the European Prospective Investigation into Cancer and Nutrition (EPIC)," *Public Health Nutrition* 5, no. 6B (December 2002): 1329–45, www.ncbi.nlm.nih.gov/pubmed/12639236.

61. U.S. Department of Agriculture, "What We Eat in America," http://www.ars.usda.gov/News/docs.htm?docid=13793

62. R. D. Mattes and R. V. Considine, "Oral Processing Effort, Appetite and Acute Energy Intake in Lean and Obese Adults," *Physiology & Behavior* 120 (August 15, 2013): 173–81.

63. M. M. Hetherington and M. F. Regan, "Effects of Chewing Gum on Short-Term Appetite Regulation in Moderately Restrained Eaters," *Appetite* 57, no. 2 (October 2011): 475–82.

64. "Calories Burned in 30 Minutes for People of Three Different Weights," Harvard Health Publications, July 1, 2004, www.health.harvard.edu/diet-and-weight-loss/calories-burned-in-30-minutes-of-leisure-and-routine-activities.

65. J. E. Flood and B. J. Rolls, "Soup Preloads in a Variety of Forms Reduce Meal Energy Intake," *Appetite* 49, no. 3 (November 2007): 626–34, www.ncbi.nlm.nih.gov/pubmed/17574705.

INDEX